WALKING FINGERS

Walking Fingers

The Story of Polio and
Those Who Lived with It

EDITED BY

Sally Aitken, Helen D'Orazio
& Stewart Valin

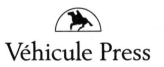

Véhicule Press

Published with the generous assistance of The Canada Council for the Arts, the Book Publishing Industry Development Program of the Department of Canadian Heritage, and the Société de développement des entreprises culturelles du Québec (SODEC).

The publisher wishes to also thank Polio Québec for its support of this book.

"Poliomyelitis" by Pierrette Caron is translated from *L'Histoire vécue de la polio au Québec* published by Carte Blanche.
"My Experience of Polio" by Victor-Lévy Beaulieu, a translation of a reminiscence written by him shortly after he contracted polio in August 1964, is reprinted by permission of the author.
Thank you to the following who provided photographs: Christopher Rutty, Polio Canada, Shriners Hospital (Montreal), the Hospital for Sick Children (Toronto), Aventis Pasteur Limited Archives, Rotary International Archives

Cover design: J.W. Stewart
Front cover: Ten-year-old Reine Bélanger, 1946. She's using a walker made by a metalworker based on a picture seen in an American magazine.
Set in Adobe Minion by Simon Garamond
Printed by AGMV-Marquis Inc.

NATIONAL LIBRARY OF CANADA CATALOGUING IN PUBLICATION

Walking fingers : the story of polio and those who lived with it / edited by Sally Aitken, Helen D'Orazio, and Stewart Valin.

Includes bibliographical references and index.
ISBN 1-55065-180-3

1. Poliomyelitis—Patients—Canada—Biography. 2. Poliomyelitis—Canada—History. I. Aitken, Sally II. D'Orazio, Helen III. Valin, Stewart

RC181.C2W34 2004   361.1'96853'0092   C2004-00005-5

Véhicule Press
www.vehiculepress.com

CANADIAN DISTRIBUTION
LitDistCo Distribution, 100 Armstrong Avenue,
Georgetown, Ontario L7G5S4 / 800.591.6250 / orders@litdistco.ca

U.S. DISTRIBUTION
Independent Publishers Group (IPG)
814 North Franklin Street, Chicago, Illinois 60610
800.888.4741 / frontdesk@ipgbook.com

Printed in Canada

To all those whose lives were cut short by polio, and to the doctors, nurses, physiotherapists, teachers, bus drivers, friends, and families who helped—and are helping—polio survivors lead full and productive lives.

Contents

Three

Polio as Experienced by Family, Friends, and the Community

Four

Teachers, Doctors, Nurses, and Volunteers

Five

Foreword

RICHARD CRUESS, M.D.

IN THE SUMMER OF 1951, between graduation from university and beginning medical school, I suffered from poliomyelitis while on vacation in rural Ontario. I spent time in a small community hospital and was fortunate enough to escape the paralyzing effects. Polio, however, did catch my attention in medical school; I made the decision to become an orthopedic surgeon during my first rotation on that specialty because of the presence of post-polio paralysis as a major problem in those pre-Salk days. I was impressed with the dedicated medical team-treatment of patients, with the motivation of the patients, particularly the children, and with the real opportunity to assist people to function better in everyday living. At the time of my training somewhere between a third and a half of our efforts were spent dealing with the consequences of polio, and this continued during my early years of practice at the Shriners Hospital for Children in Montreal.

It is difficult for recent generations to imagine the fear which "infantile paralysis" or poliomyelitis engendered half a century ago. Epidemics developed throughout the world, generally during the summer months, and struck people without warning. For many years it proved very difficult for organized medicine to address the challenge in any logical or coherent fashion. This was of course because the cause was little understood, and consequently both prevention and therapy were not based upon a scientific understanding of the problem. The cause of polio was known since the first isolation of the polio virus in 1908, although there was confusion about how it spread from person to person until the 1940s. As public health data became available, it became apparent that, at least in temperate climates, summer months were the high risk period; the data also revealed an association with close contact with crowds, suggesting a person-to-person, probably by droplet, form of transmission. It also seemed that those from higher socioeconomic groups were at greater risk. Early on it was postulated that exposure at a sub-clinical level leading to immunity probably took place where people lived in closer quarters with poorer hygiene.

The end result was that everywhere parents attempted to protect their children by avoiding crowds and swimming pools, and by carrying out other elementary public health measures. The fact that Franklin D. Roosevelt contracted polio in 1921 while on Campobello Island in the Bay of Fundy indicated that these means were, in actual fact, quite ineffective.

The management of the disease itself was on somewhat more solid ground. The treatment of the acute phase developed slowly; it was revolutionized by the advent in the 1920s of assisted respiration (the iron lung) that tided over patients who might otherwise have not survived their respiratory paralysis.

The prevention of deformities and attempts to maintain muscle strength were epitomized in Sister Elizabeth Kenny's approach, which also assured caring and compassion because of the close bond between the therapist and the patient. ("Sister" is the British title for head nurse). Finally, orthopedic surgery was actually quite effective in maximizing function once the disease had run its course and the pattern of paralysis was established. Braces were used to both prevent deformity and to stabilize the trunk and limbs when active muscle power was absent. Because the patterns of paralysis were quite variable, paralyzing some muscles in a given limb while sparing others, there was an opportunity to carry out reconstructive surgery in which the surviving muscles would be transferred in order to maximize function.

Everyone who was associated with treating people with polio was struck with their patients' desire to return to an active life. This was certainly true with the children, who comprised the most common age group. Because the disease struck individuals who had previously been physically normal, most polio patients had a self-image of functioning in society and desired to return to that state. This was in contradistinction to many other children who were paralyzed from birth, who were often mentally retarded. They rarely exhibited the same level of motivation witnessed in patients with post-polio paralysis.

The development of the Salk and Sabin vaccines was to most of us somewhere between magic and the answer to oft-repeated prayers. The virus that caused the disease was identified when microbiology introduced the techniques of modern virology in 1908. It became possible to contemplate the eradication of poliomyelitis through immunization. In developed societies we are close to achieving this. There are, however, many underdeveloped areas where vaccination programs are still difficult to organize. Nonetheless, throughout the world the scourge of infantile paralysis has been greatly lessened. The United Nations and Rotary International have set the year 2005 as their target date for global wild virus (polio) extinction.

The disease is still important to understand. Because of the reality of modern travel, both acute poliomyelitis and patients suffering from paralysis as a result of a disease acquired elsewhere, appear in western cities. In addition, the recognition of the post-polio syndrome has reawakened interest in the disease and made us realize that even those patients who acquired their paralysis many years ago still require care and compassion.

Richard Cruess was Dean of Medicine, McGill University, 1981-1995

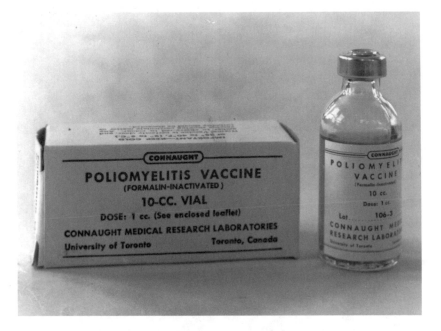

Salk vaccine vial and package, Connaught Medical Research Laboratories,
University of Toronto, 1959.
Aventis Pasteur Limited Archives.

Preface

SALLY AITKEN

IN 1996 A PUBLISHER mailed me *Polio's Legacy* by the American doctor Edmund J. Sass, and asked me to review the book. It didn't take long to realize that this was not only an opportunity to help Dr. Sass (whom I'd never heard of), but also one that might open some yet-to-be revealed door. I loved his book and told him so, and he suggested something similar could be done for Canada. We all thank you for the idea, Dr. Sass.

At the time, I was interested in seeing material about polio in French. Without any writing experience, or knowing how the project was going to come to fruition, Pierrette Caron and I started accumulating and taping over a hundred interviews with people who have had polio or were connected with polio through family or profession. With the invaluable help of Gilles Fournier, *Histoire vécu de la Polio au Québec* was published in 2000 by Carte Blanche, sponsored by Polio Quebec Association, and distributed by Fides. Sales were good and so was the feedback.

People asked the obvious question, "When are you going to translate the book?" My opinion was that an English version would have to have national appeal, and would therefore require new material and a publisher whose distribution network went far beyond Quebec. We thank Phillip Cercone of McGill-Queen's University Press for directing us to Simon Dardick of Véhicule Press. We also thank Marilynn Vanderstay for her encouragement, expertise and advice, and Polio Quebec for its moral and financial support.

It was the existence of Polio Quebec that catalyzed the awareness that such a book could inspire people challenged by disabilities and give tangible recognition to their achievements.

Polio Quebec Association grew from the original work begun by Sieglinde Stieda and the late Monique Grégoire in 1984. The Association became legally constituted on October 14, 1986 as the Quebec Post-Polio Syndrome Association (Association québécoise du syndrome post-polio). In September 1990, the Association applied for a name change and became the Polio Quebec Association (Association Polio Québec). The Association's mission is to provide support and information to those who had polio and to foster public awareness of all aspects of the disease, including prevention.

We are particularly grateful to Sieglinde Stieda, the late Monique Grégoire, Claire and Claude Mercier, and the late Joyce Jarrett, without whom polio survivors in Quebec would not have been brought together in what was to become the Polio Quebec Association. Polio Quebec assisted in the creation of this book.

The editors hope that you will enjoy this collection of polio histories told mostly through voices of those who have lived with the disease. We would like to acknowledge all those who told their stories and to thank them for sharing their memories of how polio affected their lives—memories that for many were expressed for the first time.

Selecting what should be included in this collection of life's challenges was by far the most difficult part of the editing process. To have included all the stories we had would have resulted in an unwieldy tome, too heavy for polio hands to hold!

This book differs from its French counterpart. In addition to translations of a few stories from *Histoire vécue de la polio au Québec*, there are new stories and updated information about polio. (The stories in Part Two are arranged in chronological order relating to the date when the individual contracted polio.) I am sure some readers will recognize in these narratives their struggles with polio and their successes.

My fellow editors Helen D'Orazio and Stewart Valin and I hope this book will open windows of personal and professional understanding about polio and its effects. It honours the strength, courage, and fortitude of the victims of polio and their champions.

One

Polio, Its Cure, and the Post-Polio Syndrome

Poliomyelitis – A History

PIERRETTE CARON

POLIOMYELITIS IS NOT an illness of the twentieth century. Far from it. A bas-relief dating back to 1600 B.C. in Copenhagen shows a man with a withered leg, obviously a result of his having contracted polio. However the first written mention of poliomyelitis was in Germany in 1840.[1] America became aware of it in Boston in 1893.

Poliomyelitis was called infantile paralysis for a long time because the virus seemed to attack children under ten. It was also called the Heine-Medin sickness, named after Jacob Heine and Oskar Medin. Heine was a German orthopedist who observed that polio was related to damage to motor neurons in the anterior horn cells of the spinal cord, from which voluntary muscles were controlled. Medin was a Swedish pediatrician who in 1890, following Sweden's first polio epidemic, undertook a study that attracted worldwide attention. In 1884 polio had been recognized as an infectious disease.[2] In 1907 a group of Scandinavians from the medical community determined that polio entered the body through the blood. In 1908 the polio virus was isolated by Karl Landsteiner in Vienna. Swedish researchers pioneered understanding of the natural epidemiology of polio during the period 1905 to 1910, although their results were not widely recognized at the time. In 1945 it was discovered that there were three different types of polio.

THE POSITIVE AND THE PUZZLING

Paralytic polio is an inflammation of the grey matter in the spinal cord[3] with a concomitant destruction of the affected person's motor neurons by one of the three types of polio viruses. In the majority of cases, the virus causes a mere gastro-intestinal episode, akin to summer flu and is often mistaken for it. Although no one has ever been able to determine exactly what route the virus takes, a number of studies support the hypothesis that it is spread by direct contact with a person already infected, entering the gastro-intestinal tract through the mouth. This can happen by using a contaminated table napkin or handling the soiled diaper of a child who has recently been vaccinated by the Sabin method with the live virus. Water, food, and other matter may harbour the virus. Only one case in a hundred will develop a paralysis because the person struck by the same virus as ninety-nine others simply didn't have the necessary antibodies to fight it off and is more receptive to a polio assault on the nervous system.[4]

The first symptoms of poliomyelitis are pain in the back, limbs, and the trunk, along with headaches, a high fever, shivering, occasionally nausea, a stiff neck, weakness, and extreme fatigue. In brief, the symptoms are so similar to flu that they can be confused and delay an accurate diagnosis, given that paralysis doesn't appear immediately. The incontrovertible test to confirm polio, as many of its victims will remember, was the lumbar puncture. Unfortunately, by the time this was administered it was usually too late. Harm had been done. We must remember that there were no other specific tests to assist doctors in making an early diagnosis; many conditions had similar symptoms.

There are practically no statistics on the occurrence of polio prior to 1900. We know it was endemic in most countries. Infants exposed to the virus might get mild infections which in many cases actually immunized them against the disease. Paralytic complications were rare until improved hygiene around 1900 delayed exposure, especially in the northern European countries, the United States, and Canada, and among the middle and upper classes.

Poliomyelitis was one of the most puzzling infectious diseases for the medical community.[5] It could come upon a person unnoticed and leave that person visibly unaffected, or it could irrevocably handicap a person in a couple of days, even a couple of hours. Swimming pools[6] and tonsillectomies were to be avoided during epidemic years.[7] An explanation as to why some people were affected and others not could also be attributed to a weakened immune system, or even fatigue.

The incidence of polio usually peaked at the end of summer, tapering off by the end of the autumn season. This however did not preclude the possibility of getting polio at any time of the year. It is therefore plausible to think that the climate has an influence on polio, because people come together more in the summer, whereas people are more stay-at-homes in the cold weather. This idea, however, is discredited by a polio epidemic that struck during the coldest of winter months in 1948-49 around Chesterfield Inlet near the western shore of Hudson Bay in the Northwest Territories.[8] Science just doesn't always fathom these mysteries.

THERAPEUTIC APPROACHES
Medical literature cites numerous therapeutic approaches for the treatment of poliomyelitis: convalescent serum, i.e., serum from the recovered polio cases, ultraviolet treatment, diathermy, application of galvanic currents, and physiotherapy. The most revolutionary method, however, was the Sister Kenny

treatment with hot packs.

Elizabeth Kenny, an Australian, became interested in polio as far back as 1911.[9] The scientific world doubted her procedure of treating polio with heated moist hot material known as hot packs, but it was forced to acknowledge the good results, especially when treatment was started in the earliest possible stages of contracting the disease. The primary objective of this treatment was to relieve muscle spasm, the cause of pain and muscle contraction, leading ultimately to deformities. Sister Kenny's treatment consisted of wrapping all the affected muscles in hot and moist blankets every two hours, twelve hours a day, until the spasms were relieved, a minimum of ten days. This procedure replaced the immobilization of polio patients in plaster casts, a treatment that prevailed up until about 1940 and often left patients with contracted and atrophied muscles, a condition which was next to impossible to correct.

Convalescent serum, or serotherapy as it was commonly called, was used for the first time in France in 1915.[10] It was an essential part of treating polio for a number of years, but to be effective it had to be administered in the pre-paralytic phase. It was therefore essential that there be an early diagnosis, which was difficult for the majority because the economic crisis which ravaged the 1930s prevented people from calling for medical help, knowing they wouldn't be able to assume the cost of a professional visit, even though the serum was given out at no cost by most provincial governments in this period. These were pre-Medicare days. Serotherapy consisted of giving a recently diagnosed polio patient the blood of a recovered patient who would have sufficient antibodies to fight against the virus at work in the new patient. This treatment was very popular in Europe. In the 1930s in North America there was considerable scepticism, and it was soon shown that the serum was not only innocuous but also ineffective. Nonetheless, the increase of poliomyelitis cases during this period led provincial governments to subscribe to this therapeutic measure despite its dubious results, in a desperate effort to be seen to be trying to wipe out this disease across Canada. The Great Depression was a period in history when people needed to feel their government was doing something about a disease that was affecting so many on a personal, social, and economic level. Since there was nothing else to offer, the serum continued to be used well into the 1940s.

Despite everything, these polio epidemics had some positive results. Without any doubt, they had an enormous impact on the evolution of rehabilitation medicine (physiatry). Quebec's pioneer in this field was Dr. Gustave Gingras, founder of the Institut de Réadaptation de Montréal. The principles established nearly fifty years ago to help polio victims recover residual muscle function are still used today to rehabilitate those who have had head injuries, spinal cord injuries, cerebro-vascular accidents (strokes), or a degenerative disease.

Support for Families

After the first major poliomyelitis epidemic in Canada in 1927, federal and provincial governments, particularly those of Ontario, Manitoba, and Saskatchewan, began prevention programs, offering free treatment and hospital services for all victims. Alberta was the first province to offer special support for polio patients, opening a polio hospital in 1928 and enacting the Polio Sufferers Act in 1938.

The illness preoccupied government authorities and the medical community alike. Quebec limited itself to applying the Public Assistance Law already in place. In that period in Quebec, help for those with restricted incomes was given by the religious orders that administered most of the French hospitals, and by philanthropic associations both English and French— Rotary Clubs, the Kiwanians, and the Lions Clubs. In 1930, with help from the Lions Club, Madame M.A. Daigle started the Société de secours aux enfants infirmes de la province de Québec, known today as the Société pour les enfants handicapés du Québec. It was followed by the Canadian Red Cross and the March of Dimes. A large number of children were left paralyzed or had to wear braces for many years or had to undergo treatment as outpatients. For countless families, the Société de secours aux enfants infirmes provided transport for children to the Montreal hospitals and assumed the costs of braces and orthopedic boots as well as crutches, which of course had to be changed frequently as the child grew. In addition, the Boards of Directors of certain hospitals, aware of the costs polio placed upon a family that had been affected, voluntarily lowered the hospital fee, and the health authorities of the time enlarged the admissibility criteria for public assistance for numerous families.[11] The Shriners Hospital in Montreal was particularly involved. It financed all hospital costs, including medical, orthopedic appliances, and other expenses incurred by polio victims not only in Montreal, but also throughout Quebec as well as New Brunswick and Ontario.

The Situation in the Hospitals

Cooperation was established among the hospitals across Canada. Thus, in 1941 when a serious epidemic burst onto the New Brunswick scene, their provincial government sought the advice of the Montreal Children's Hospital, which assigned a member of its personnel, a British physiotherapist Kathleen Walker,[12] to help them out. At this time in Quebec there did not exist any training programs for physiotherapists. Only after the war did physiotherapy become

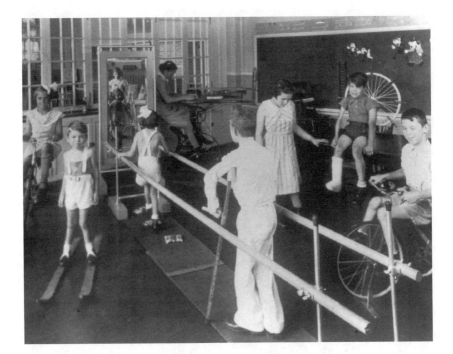

"A large number of children were left paralyzed or had to wear braces for many years or had to undergo treatment as outpatients."
Shriners Hospital, Montreal.

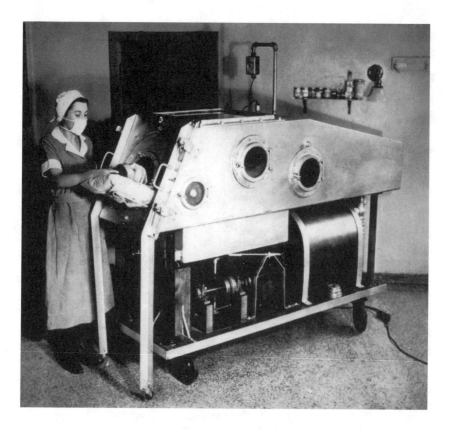

The iron lung.
"This cylindrical cage, which allowed the patient to breathe and, in many cases, to survive, was a miraculous technological gadget for those imprisoned within it for a number of weeks or months, if not for the rest of their lives."
The Hospital for Sick Children (Toronto), Hospital Archives.

a degree course. Therapists trained in Europe were greatly in demand, but they were scarce. In 1946, it was Quebec that was the most seriously affected by polio; the Department of Veterans Affairs sent a physiotherapist to Ste. Justine Hospital and the Canadian Association of Physiotherapists sent two for two months requiring Ste. Justine to be insured should one of their physios succumb to polio because they were of a vulnerable age.[13]

During the major epidemics in the period 1940-1950, some hospitals were turned into special treatment centres for poliomyelitis. Nursing and medical staff was inadequate, given the enormity of the situation, and they had to work countless overtime hours. To compensate, the Minister of National Revenue, Dr. McCann, in a letter dated September 4, 1946, decreed that income tax not be deducted from salaries for the additional hours worked by nurses looking after cases of infantile paralysis.[14]

The overwhelmed hospitals would line up dozens of beds in large rooms or wards. Some of the patients were hundreds of miles from home and felt literally abandoned. The caregivers were preoccupied with treating the paralysis and had little time for the emotional upheaval the young patient was experiencing. There are many examples of the long-term effect this had on some patients, while others would forget their families completely and consider the hospital as their home—a place where they were treated affectionately by the nurses and the nuns.

Wherever there was an outbreak of polio, the hospitals would find themselves short of staff and medical equipment. Consequently, in 1939, the technical staff of Ste. Justine Hospital in Montreal, for instance, manufactured their own iron lungs, also called pulmometers or lung-respirators.[15] Organizations like the Catholic Diocesan Action Committee enlarged its social mission and made public appeals for volunteers which were directed to women's organizations. Help was needed especially around mealtime because many polio victims had lost the use of their arms.

INCIDENCE OF POLIO

In 1946 Quebec experienced its most devastating year with 1,612 victims, and 115 deaths. This accounted for more than half of all the cases reported throughout Canada that year. Montreal was the most severely affected, with 625 cases and 25 deaths. This was also the case in 1931. Between 1927 and 1953, poliomyelitis tended to increase not only in incidences, but also in severity. In Canada the largest epidemic was in 1953, with 8,818 recorded cases, of whom 401 died. In 1953 it was a greater cause of death in Canada than tuberculosis.[16] It is estimated that 50 percent of those who were affected by the poliovirus recovered completely, 29 percent were left with muscular weakness, 18 percent were permanently incapacitated, and 3 percent did not survive.[17] Between 1927 and 1962 there were 50,000 cases reported throughout Canada; 4240 people died of the disease in that period.

The population explosion following World War II coincided with the largest polio epidemics in Canada, sowing panic among parents. Between 1945 and 1952 alone, the number of cases tripled compared to the average in the years 1924-1944. In 1946, for example, the public was asked to be calm because the hospitals were already overflowing with polio cases, and they kept coming. In addition, anxious parents were calling hospitals and doctors incessantly.

The most terrifying image that this illness evoked was paradoxically not that of death, but that of the iron lung. This cylindrical cage, which allowed the patient to breathe and, in many cases, to survive, was a miraculous technological gadget for those imprisoned within it for a number of weeks or months, if not for the rest of their lives. The pulmonary respirator's role was to supplant respiratory deficiency by expanding and contracting the thoracic cage. Philip Drinker put the first one together in 1928 at Harvard University. It was brought to Canada by the Toronto Children's Hospital two years later. It was the only such apparatus in Canada until 1937.[18] Before this time all those who had bulbar polio died.

In 1947 poliomyelitis, instead of restricting itself to the young, began affecting an increasing number of adolescents and adults. They were particularly vulnerable to Type III of the poliovirus. The reason was that during and following World War II there was a lot of national and international travel that exposed people to the poliovirus who had not built up an immunity. Their immune systems could not respond effectively to it.

Another factor was the post-war baby boom. There were lots of young parents with several children living mostly in new subdivisions that were relatively isolated from the poliovirus. However, once the virus entered these communities it spread quickly among the babies and to their parents, many of whom who were relatively young and had never been exposed to it. The poliovirus attacked the anterior horn cells of the spinal cord or lower brain stem. The location and degree of damage the virus did there determined the location and severity of its paralytic effects. It could, in addition to affecting one or more limbs, paralyze the thoracic cage, which would cause a problem with swallowing as well as respiratory distress, requiring the use of an iron lung.[19] In the last big epidemic of 1959, there were 17 recorded cases of people over forty and 28.6 percent of all those struck were over twenty years old. Worthy of note also is that out of the 1,171 polios reported that year, 5 percent had been vaccinated, 10 percent were in the process of being vaccinated, and 85 percent had received no protection at all against poliomyelitis.[20]

Stastistical Table
Number of cases declared in Canada by province - 1927-1962[18]

(1927-1956: all declared cases)
1957-1962*: (paralytic cases only)

Year	CAN	BC	ALB	SASK	MAN.	ONT	QC	NB	NS	PEI	NWT
1927	609	182	313	8	6	52	14	16	26	0	
1928	787	102	93	26	434	85	37	5	10	0	
1929	707	43	45	59	58	480	90	5	3	4	
1930	1027	34	144	70	45	671	35	1	28	4	
1931	1342	42	23	5	15	161	1077	6	13	0	
1932	956	5	35	6	7	175	769	13	4	2	
1933	255	5	31	28	7	53	124	5	2	0	
1934	520	32	11	12	10	325	115	3	10	1	
1935	363	20	152	21	24	108	32	3	2	1	
1936	978	27	16	77	525	208	122	3	0	0	
1937	3905	26	167	519	267	2546	172	164	43	1	
1938	577	43	104	34	160	160	54	17	5	0	
1939	359	1	24	11	26	216	59	2	20	0	
1940	192	5	2	9	18	91	64	1	2	0	
1941	1881	58	166	598	969	143	48	419	19	0	
1942	687	47	8	15	72	92	152	135	162	3	
1943	327	8	20	37	38	81	113	18	9	3	
1944	722	19	97	17	99	337	47	85	20	1	
1945	384	52	14	20	24	184	57	7	26	0	
1946	2527	21	68	37	48	518	1612	94	49	80	
1947	2291	312	82	277	587	796	144	20	71	2	
1948	1168	125	359	84	142	372	46	10	29	1	
1949	2458	229	129	111	119	1138	587	40	85	0	20
1950	911	76	138	120	22	376	77	15	17	67	3
1951	2568	92	59	92	55	1701	274	51	216	23	5
1952	4755	596	740	1205	839	705	125	427	57	57	4
1953	8878	797	1472	1202	2317	2239	488	88	31	11	233
1954	2390	217	523	197	114	250	786	61	137	83	22
1955	1021	230	215	72	33	169	122	39	115	11	15
1956	600	84	76	21	22	193	152	24	20	4	4
1957*	182	26	31	20	8	54	37	5	0	0	1
1958*	249	12	22	1	107	20	79	4	0	0	4
1959*	1886	132	83	46	26	200	1171	62	9	7	139
1960*	909	165	201	56	13	39	284	92	9	1	49
1961*	188	6	26	7	0	23	115	1	1	0	9
1962*	89	2	5	3	4	19	56	1	1	0	0
Total	49 711	3873	5694	4584	7260	14 981	9336	1942	1251	367	508

When the disease began attacking adults, a new socio-economic problem was created. There were fathers functioning as breadwinners who were no longer able to work, and mothers with lots of children; some were pregnant and had to come to term in an iron lung. The baby might be born healthy, but some were premature and others miscarried. Imagine a paralyzed mother who had to leave her young children at home or a father deprived of his income because of a long hospitalization. This translated into a serious financial crisis for many.

Around 1949 insurance companies began offering policies for polio-myelitis, which created a real problem for actuaries who had to calculate the risks in the face of the unpredictability of the seriousness of polio or the colossal expenses that it might entail. These insurance plans sold well, but since many companies suffered heavy losses, in the peak year of 1953, when Canada reported an unprecedented number of polio cases—8,878[21]—the sale of policies covering polio was discontinued.[22]

Today: Post-Polio Syndrome

By the middle of the 1960s poliomyelitis was for the most part eradicated from North America—at least we believed this to be so. We no longer spoke of it in terms of an illness, but rather about the vaccine. The medical world, the general population, and even those affected by polio were all persuaded that once over the rehabilitation period, after having achieved a certain functional recovery plateau, everyone's condition would remain more or less stable, apart from the natural aging process.

But at the end of the 1970s alarming new difficulties were reported by those who had had polio decades ago. French medical literature had identified this problem way back in 1875,[23] but as often happens in the scientific world, this was forgotten. As a result, doctors who heard these new complaints from their patients could not understand the cause. It is a well-known axiom in medicine that a syndrome that doesn't have a name cannot be treated! However, the number of people with polio complaining about new problems alerted the medical community. At the beginning of the 1980s a name was put to this ensemble of symptoms: the post-polio syndrome. Despite all the articles written about post-polio syndrome, even today many doctors know nothing about it or don't even credit its existence. Symptoms are excessive fatigue and muscular and joint pain, and most worrying, the new and progressive muscular weaknesses that creep up insidiously, sometimes triggered by a minor accident, a fall, or surgery.

Several theories have been put forward to identify the causes. The most plausible is that new weakness is a result of overuse of motor neurons that survived the destruction of neighbouring neurons by polio, and which had a heavy task imposed upon them compensating for the destroyed motor neurons. One must understand that every human being loses motor neurons with age. It is completely normal. But with polio, this diminution does not relate to age and affects those who are already weak, which explains the disproportionate muscular loss with post-polio compared to the natural loss that comes with aging.

Most of those who got poliomyelitis when young learned to cope and got on with their lives, considering themselves perhaps limited, but not handicapped. This makes accepting new weaknesses and a changed way of life more difficult; it's as if the mourning of abilities lost thirty or forty years ago was happening now.

Is there a treatment? As in all chronic conditions, the medical world tries to relieve the symptoms of pain and fatigue and tries to improve the muscular function enough in order to give the patient back an acceptable quality of life. To do this, appliances like braces as well as changing life patterns must be considered. To remain fit physically and psychologically, keeping active is strongly recommended. An exercise program, moderate for some, a little more vigorous for others, supervised by a professional, is very important.

No history of polio would be complete without giving tribute to the untiring devotion of the parents of the children affected by poliomyelitis. Almost without exception the responsibility of post-hospital care fell upon the mothers; their efforts on their children's behalf were often heroic. Many survivors remember the hours spent every day, often for years, by their mothers, at times their fathers, helping them do stretching, flexibility, and strengthening exercises. Because they had to work for many years recouping their muscular strength, old "polios" often developed a special knowledge of their bodies, a relationship one doesn't necessarily find in the population at large. For some, exercise became a major preoccupation, for others, a life habit. When a therapist recommended doing a certain movement ten times twice a day to strengthen a muscle, the patient would do it thirty times, three times a day. This visceral compulsion always to go beyond the limit carries over into other facets of survivors' lives, which is why we often find polio survivors first in their class and top performers in the workplace.

Another reality, particularly present in predominantly Catholic Quebec during the epidemic years, was the belief in miracles. Many parents would take their polio-affected child to St. Joseph's Oratory in Montreal, to the sanctuaries at Ste. Anne de Beaupré or to Notre-Dame-du-Cap. Some would consult a healer hoping for a miracle that would wipe out all traces of paralysis, lengthen the withered limb, or reshape deformities. But Brother André, the good Saint Anne, and Notre Dame were never there. While miracles were perhaps not tangible, you will find while reading about the experiences many had with polio, that most of them tell a story full of combat and victory. Debilitating paralysis to begin with was usually followed by a recovery period, ranging from a partial to a visibly complete recovery. Thanks to their determination and ingenuity those who were left with permanent lameness, no matter how severe, learned to compensate for their motor deficits. This allowed them to lead an active life, which was usually satisfying and very often prosperous.

It is certain that no one with polio would say twenty, thirty, or forty years after the acute phase of poliomyelitis that he or she is ill. Compared to the Spanish flu which took the lives of thousands in 1918-1919, or tuberculosis, cancer, or heart disease, which however tragic could pass unnoticed if the person or those around him didn't speak of the illness, poliomyelitis had something unique. It left some with a permanent lameness and it was visible. With the growing number of cases that accrued following every epidemic, society found itself with a new minority, the survivors of poliomyelitis. It is from this visibly handicapped group whose numbers kept increasing right up until the beginning of the 1960s, that the movement for the rights of handicapped persons was born, a movement which permitted everyone, whatever his or her physical or intellectual limitations, to be considered a citizen like all others, with rights and prerogatives appropriate to his or her situation.

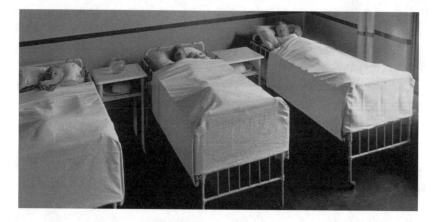

"Overwhelmed hospitals would line up dozens of beds in large rooms or wards. Some of the patients were hundreds of miles from home and felt literally abandoned."
The Hospital for Sick Children (Toronto), Hospital Archives.

Sister Kenny: Although Untrained, She Got Results

HELEN D'ORAZIO

SISTER ELIZABETH KENNY will be long remembered as a polio crusader. She stood firm in her beliefs about treating polio patients. Before her, some patients could only dream about walking again because splinting and immobility were the main options practiced by the medical community. Sister Kenny advocated a more active approach for treating polio-ravaged muscles and, for some, walking again as well as regaining use of previously paralyzed muscles became a reality.

Elizabeth "Liza" Kenny grew up in bush houses in Australia, where she was born in 1880. She had some schooling from family members. Even as a child she had enjoyed playing nurse with her doll; this was at a time when diseases such as diphtheria, pneumonia, scarlet fever, and smallpox were prevalent.[24]

After learning much about muscle structure from the local doctor, Dr. McDonnell, Liza rigged up a wooden man with pulleys and strings to show her frail brother Willie how muscles work.

She traveled from village to village caring for the sick. Her first encounter with polio was in 1911 when she came upon a two-year-old girl whose body was twisted and deformed and who was unable to move. Amy screamed in pain as Liza gently tried straightening her arm and leg. She had never seen this before. She consulted Dr. McDonnell by telegram. He replied "Infantile paralysis. No known treatment. Do the best you can with the symptoms presenting themselves."[25] She applied hot moist cloths around the affected limbs for many hours. This helped relax the muscles and enabled her to straighten the limbs. Liza treated six other patients with the same methods and all recovered without paralysis.

World War I prevented her from continuing her bush nursing. She became a military nurse, now known as Sister Kenny. She worked on hospital ships bringing the injured back to Australia. She was discharged because of a heart condition and returned to bush nursing, and thus began her crusade for polio patients.

She opened her first polio clinic in an Australian back yard in 1932. Money she had received from inventing a stretcher to help transport patients was used to finance the clinic. Polio treatment hadn't changed much since her first patient, Amy. There wasn't much hope for polio victims. They were still being splinted and immobilized, which only caused more deformity and muscle atrophy. Sister Kenny called these twisted bodies living corpses.[26]

The medical community believed that polio was a disease of the central nervous system and healthy muscles were causing deformities by pulling on the weak ones affected by the poliovirus.

Sister Kenny believed from her experience that polio was a muscle disease and that spasms shortened and tightened the muscles, causing pain. Hot moist towels on affected muscles and gentle stretching when they relaxed got her results. She knew she could work with any muscle that had a flicker of movement in it.[27] She was a very stubborn, not very diplomatic woman who insisted on using only her methods. Although most medical experts would have nothing to do with her unscientific approach, some doctors believed her treatments helped and sent their patients to her.

Sister Kenny came to Canada during the epidemic of 1941 in Manitoba. At the time there was no active treatment for polio until after two to three weeks of isolation and immobilization. She stressed the importance of implementing her methods during the acute phase. Within one year a committee in Ottawa concluded that Sister Kenny's method was as good as and probably better than splinting.[28] Various doctors, including Dr. Betty Fraser of Montreal's Children's Memorial Hospital, as well as nurses and physio-therapists were sent to Kenny clinics in the early 1940s to learn the Kenny method. In the late summer of 1942 Montreal experienced another polio epidemic. Ninety-five acute cases of polio were admitted to the Children's.[29]

Sister Kenny visited the Children's Memorial Hospital in Montreal in June 1943. It was a well-publicized and anticipated event. Andee Millstock, who remembers being scalded from the hot packs, was a thirteen-year-old stricken with polio at the time. She was chosen for a demonstration. Many doctors, nurses, and physiotherapists were in the room to watch the impressive Sister Kenny in action.

The Kenny concept of polio was a new approach to its diagnosis and treatment. Sister Kenny triggered research into neuromuscular physiology and anatomy. A large part of her contribution was her stubborn refusal to accept the inevitability of crippling at a time when it was generally accepted. She gave hope. Seeing patients in casts, she not only knew it was wrong, it was defeatist. She was not a scientist; she was a crusader. The Kenny method shifted attention away from splints to active hospital treatment. Responsibility for long-term treatment also shifted from home to hospital, and from physicians and parents to nurses and physiotherapists.[30]

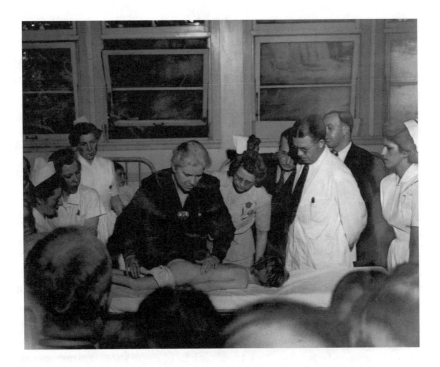

Sister Kenny (centre) at the Children's Memorial Hospital, Montreal, June 1943, examining Sally (Drysdale) Aitken. Among the attending physicians are Dr. Struthers and Dr. Goldbloom. *News Pictures of Canada.*

Post-Polio Syndrome

DARIA A. TROJAN, M.D., M.SC.

ACUTE PARALYTIC POLIOMYELITIS is now a preventable disease due to the introduction of effective vaccination in the 1950s. Vaccination efforts have been so successful that wild-type poliomyelitis has been eliminated in the Western hemisphere in the last decade, and the number of cases worldwide continues to decline.[32] Because of this, polio is a forgotten and conquered disease for many, including the medical community. However, many individuals who have survived this illness are alive today. In 1987, it was estimated that there were 640,000 people who had recovered from paralytic polio in the United States.[33] It has become increasingly recognized over the last few decades that these individuals' polio symptoms are, unfortunately, not indefinitely stable, but that many may develop new difficulties related to polio later in life.[34] This recognition came primarily as a result of the persistent effort of the patients who eventually convinced the medical community that they were indeed experiencing a new disorder.[35]

"Post-polio syndrome" has been the term most frequently used to describe these new difficulties. The main clinical features of this syndrome are a new persistent muscular weakness or muscular fatigue (reduced endurance) in people who have recovered from paralytic polio.[36] A bewildering variety of other symptoms can also occur, including generalized fatigue, muscle and joint pain, new muscular atrophy (loss of muscle bulk), breathing difficulties, swallowing difficulties, cold intolerance, muscular cramps and twitches, and joint deformities.[37, 38] The onset is usually several decades following the acute illness, and in most cases begins in mid-adulthood.[39] Studies have found that anywhere from 20 to 60 percent of people with previous paralytic polio can develop new weakness, but an even higher percentage may develop new neuromuscular complaints.[40-45]

Post-polio syndrome is considered to be a slowly progressive neuro-muscular disease.[46, 47] It is rarely fatal, but difficulties with swallowing and breathing are potentially dangerous. The symptoms of post-polio syndrome most frequently produce mobility problems. Basic activities of daily living like dressing and eating are rarely affected, but instrumental activities such as cooking, cleaning, and shopping are more commonly affected.[48]

The cause of post-polio syndrome remains poorly understood. A number of theories have been proposed;[49] the most widely accepted is that put forward by Wiechers and Hubbell[50, 51] in the 1980s (Figure 1). This theory states that new weakness and fatigue in post-polio syndrome are related to the recovery process after paralytic polio.

There are four stages in patients who have recovered from paralytic polio.

During the first stage, the acute paralytic polio phase, the poliovirus infects the spinal cord and destroys all or some of the motor nerve cells (motor neurons) that support (or innervate) a particular muscle. A motor nerve cell transmits information for muscle control from the spinal cord (and brain) to a particular muscle. Weakness or partial paralysis results when a portion of motor nerve cells which support a muscle is destroyed because the link between the spinal cord and muscle is interrupted. If all motor nerve cells supporting a particular muscle are destroyed, complete paralysis (inability to use a muscle) occurs. A motor unit is a motor nerve cell and all the muscle cells that it innervates. Normal motor units and the acute stage of polio are illustrated in the first two drawings of Figure 1.

In the second stage, or recovery phase, surviving motor nerve cells attempt to compensate for the destroyed motor nerve cells. They grow distal sprouts and form new connections to the muscle cells whose motor nerve cells were lost during the acute illness. Because of this restoration of support of muscle, the connection between the spinal cord and muscle is restored, and the ability to produce a muscle contraction returns or improves. This recovery process produces an increase in the number of muscle cells supported by a particular motor nerve cell (enlargement of motor unit size). The surviving motor nerve cells can end up supporting more muscle cells than normal, up to seven to eight times the normal amount.[52] In addition, the muscle cells that are supported by motor nerve cells can enlarge through activity or exercise, producing a further improvement in muscle strength. The third drawing in Figure 1 illustrates the recovery phase after acute paralytic polio.

The third stage is thought to be a period of stability that usually lasts several decades. Patients are stable both from the neurological and functional point of view. This stage is likely characterized by a "continuous remodeling" process. As part of this process, the sprouts of some motor nerve cells may degenerate or die off. However, new sprouts are formed by neighbouring motor nerve cells, and this restores support to these muscle cells.

The fourth stage is the post-polio syndrome phase, or a period of decline. The surviving motor nerve cells which may be supporting many more muscle cells than normal, may gradually "give out". A distal breakdown (degeneration) of overextended motor units is thought to occur. This process can produce a

Pathophysiology of Post-Poliomyelitis Syndrome

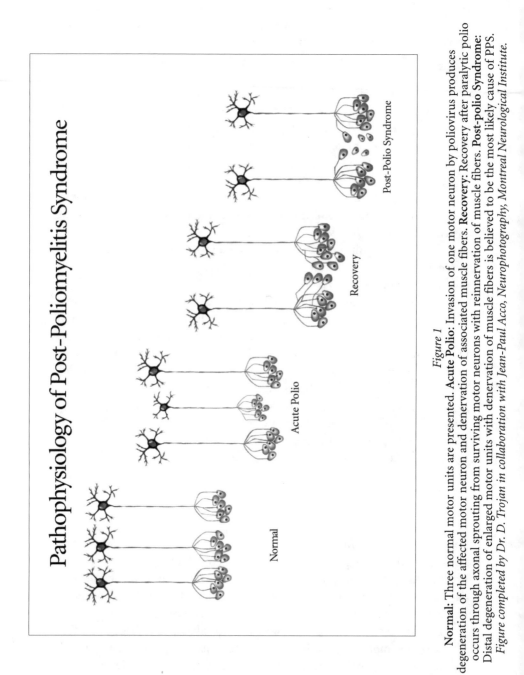

Figure 1

Normal: Three normal motor units are presented. **Acute Polio:** Invasion of one motor neuron by poliovirus produces degeneration of the affected motor neuron and denervation of associated muscle fibers. **Recovery:** Recovery after paralytic polio occurs through axonal sprouting from surviving motor neurons with reinnervation of muscle fibers. **Post-polio Syndrome:** Distal degeneration of enlarged motor units with denervation of muscle fibers is believed to be the most likely cause of PPS.
Figure completed by Dr. D. Trojan in collaboration with Jean-Paul Acco, Neurophotography, Montreal Neurological Institute.

gradual loss of sprouts, with a slow loss of support to muscle cells and resultant increased weakness. It may also produce abnormalities in the communication between the nerve and muscle (neuromuscular junction defects), with resultant muscular fatigue. The distal motor unit breakdown is illustrated in Figure 1.

There may be other contributing factors to the onset of post-polio syndrome. These can be overuse, the normal aging process, and disuse.[53, 54] Overuse has been identified as a potential cause of new weakness in people who had polio many decades ago, and should be avoided.[55-57]

However, disuse is also a well-known cause of weakness.[58] Therefore, a balance must be found for each individual. The normal aging process is associated with many changes. Aging produces a gradual loss of motor nerve cells (motor neurons), which may be especially important to people with previous polio because they have a smaller number of motor nerve cells to innervate their muscle.[59, 60] For these individuals, the natural loss of motor nerve cells may be much more noticeable.

Several studies have identified risk factors for post-polio syndrome.[61-66] A greater severity of acute paralytic polio has consistently been shown to be the most important risk factor. Other risk factors are a greater functional recovery after acute polio, a longer time since acute polio, and a greater age at presentation to clinic. Associated factors are a recent weight gain, muscle pain, especially if it is associated with exercise, and joint pain.[67]

The diagnosis of post-polio syndrome requires a confirmation of previous paralytic polio, followed by an exhaustive search for other conditions that produce similar symptoms.[68] There is no specific diagnostic test for this condition currently.[69] The symptoms of post-polio are very similar to the symptoms of many other neurological and medical disorders that occur frequently in this age group. In addition, certain disorders that occur commonly in post-polio patients such as sleep apnea, osteoporosis, and fibromyalgia should be identified and treated.[70]

Even though there is as yet no specific treatment for post-polio syndrome, many people with this disorder can benefit from an individualized management program.[71-73] Because patients can present with such a wide variety of symptoms, frequently a team of several physicians and health-care personnel is necessary.

Initially, the main thrust of the management program usually involves teaching the patient to avoid overuse. This can require education on energy conservation techniques and pacing and frequently necessitates a reduction in activity. Once the patient has learned to monitor and manage fatigue, an individualized exercise program can be introduced, under the supervision of an experienced physiotherapist. But additional exercise should be completely avoided in patients who are already very weak or fatigued.

The management program for a particular patient should be symptom-specific. The program can include interventions such as judicious exercise, avoidance of overuse, orthoses (braces), use of assistive devices (e.g., canes, crutches, wheelchairs, scooters), pacing (taking regular rest periods during any activity), weight loss, use of energy conservation techniques (e.g., sitting instead of standing, calling for home deliveries), lifestyle changes, naps or rest periods during the day to manage fatigue, improvement of sleep, and use of certain medications (primarily for pain management).[74-79] Some patients who are faced with post-polio syndrome may have great difficulty adjusting to this unexpected disability, and may need psychosocial help.

Over the last fifteen years, I have had the privilege and opportunity to care for many people who have survived this scourge of the past century. They are a unique group of individuals who not only survived a devastating illness, but truly conquered it. Many of my patients, despite great obstacles, have tried to outdo their peers in an effort to prove that they were regular members of society. To these people, the thought of a new illness related to polio later in life comes as a great shock that is difficult to accept and accommodate into their usual very active lifestyle. Successful coping with post-polio syndrome is very different than coping with acute polio. In many cases, patients must learn to conserve what they have, adapt to their new weakness and fatigue, perhaps give up some activities or perform them differently, and use new devices. Certain individuals may view asking for help or using assistive devices as a step toward dependency. However, it is important for patients to understand that by adjusting to their limitations, further deterioration can be minimized, and independence and quality of life can be preserved. This book will present some of the amazing life experiences of this courageous group of individuals. I believe we all have much to learn from them.

Two

Polio Stories

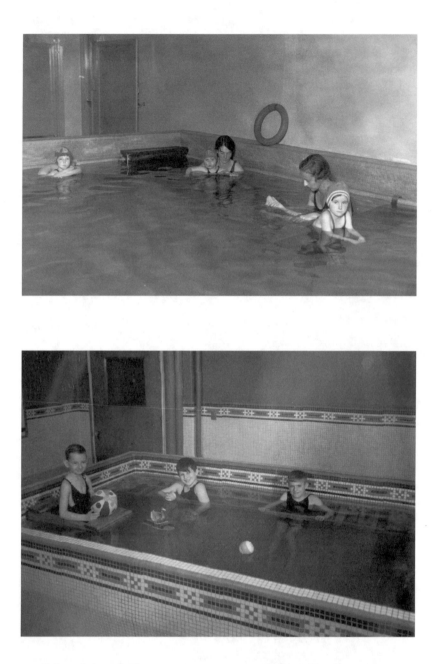

In hospitals and other treatment centres, water therapy was important.
(Top) *The Hospital for Sick Children (Toronto) Archives.*
(Bottom) *Shriners Hospital, Montreal.*

It Was a Privilege Having Polio

Tony Shorgan

I GOT POLIO IN 1923 when I was eighteen months old. Needless to say, I have no recollection of the beginning of this disease. As well, having lost my mother when I was nine years old, I don't have much information on what really happened, but apparently my parents were not aware that I had polio right away. I don't know when the diagnosis was made. I must have gone to the hospital where I had been born in Hamilton, Ontario. Health care was not government-insured at that time. I know my parents spent a fortune on my care. They had to sell our family home and never quite fully recovered financially.

My first memories go back to when I was three or four, when my family moved to Montreal. I remember numerous hospital visits over many years to the Children's Memorial Hospital where I underwent physiotherapy treatments, and also to the Montreal General Hospital, then on de la Gauchetière Street. In 1930, I was the first beneficiary of the Quebec Society for Crippled Children (now the Quebec Society for Disabled Children/la Société pour les enfants handicapés du Québec). I was examined by an orthopedic specialist, Dr. Saint-Jacques, who was practicing at Ste. Jeanne-D'Arc Hospital. He operated on me to stabilize my ankle and foot after which I wore an ankle brace for some time. I started using a cane when I was forty, and ten years later I was using two canes, probably because of my weight. I used to weigh 115 pounds; now I weigh 180 pounds.

I was the favourite of the family. My brother who is eighteen months older and my sister who is two years younger have always supported me; they felt bad for me when they saw I couldn't do as much as they could. They overprotected me, as did my mother. When my mother, who was from the Ukraine, wrote to her family, she would only talk about Tony and never the rest of the family, according to an older aunt who now lives in Canada. She wanted me to make my mark in life. She gave me special attention, and I can't say I didn't like it. I would have to check with my brother and sister to see if they felt neglected. My mother was ill for a long period of time, and I had little contact with her during her last years of life.

The polio affected mostly my left leg, leaving me with a significant weakness in my knee, ankle, and foot. I limped, but this never prevented me from following other children in all the activities appropriate at each age level. I went to Victor Doré School for one year, followed by many years at the local school. When I finished high school, because I enjoyed drawing, I studied three years at the school for fine art.

I had some bad experiences growing up, but I can't complain; when I look back, I can say my polio was almost a blessing. I would certainly not have accomplished as much if it weren't for my polio. I had some discouraging moments; for example, when I was young, I wanted to be a Scout just like my friends, but I wasn't allowed to because people were afraid I wouldn't be able to follow the others, and I didn't take this too well. Later, when I was fifteen or sixteen I felt left out because I couldn't do what the other boys and girls could; I would go to the park to watch them skate to music, while I had to sit on the sidelines.

I never had problems with how other children treated me; they would sometimes make remarks, but I always blended well with others and felt accepted. I took part in many sports, swimming for example. I would swim two miles a day, something many non-handicapped people couldn't do. I even became a qualified instructor for the Red Cross. I also skied, but actually I did more acrobatics than downhill skiing. At times I took some nasty falls. When I asked Dr. Shannon, my doctor at the Montreal Children's Hospital, about going skiing, he said, "There are enough people with fractures from skiing. You have only one good leg. Don't do such a silly thing." It was the time of the Second World War and Dr. Shannon went overseas. I took advantage of his absence to disregard his recommendations. On weekends, I would go to St. Alphonse where we had our summer cottage; I would ask my caregiver to lend me his skis. They were handcrafted skis, without a harness, and held in place with laces. Because I didn't want anyone to watch me, I would hide behind the barn and practice. At first I would take five steps and fall. I would get up and fall again. After a half-hour I managed to do the whole length of the barn.

A little while later, Maria Alida Daigle, founder and director-general of the Quebec Society for Crippled Children and my adoptive mother, bought me a pair of skis with all the necessary equipment. I started skiing in the fields of Val-David, then I ventured out onto the small hills. A few years later I was able to keep up with my friends. On top of that, I took the risk of ski jumping— not Olympic jumps, but ten- to fifteen-foot distances. I must admit I was never able to lift off with both skis; I always fell, but I never gave up. I also did a lot of horseback riding for many years, which was an excellent form of exercise for me. It is true that today my balance isn't very good, but I'm amazed when I think of everything I dared to do.

One day at the hotel a person who was less handicapped than I asked me, "Were you just skiing on the hills?" Because I had had a few to drink, I boldly lifted my pants and showed him my atrophied leg. He was stunned and said to me, "I can ski too then." The same thing happened when I was director of a swimming program at the Society's camp at St. Alphone de Rodriquez; one week after receiving my instructor's certificate from the Red Cross, I decided to display my badge on my bathing suit. I wanted to show the children that despite their limits, they could learn to swim and even become an instructor. I remember the reaction as being extraordinary. That summer everyone wanted to take swimming lessons. Because of this a publicity campaign was launched in the newspapers and approximately twenty handicapped children passed their junior Red Cross test.

During my schooling, I was sometimes invited to a social gathering in the evening, but I didn't want to go because I couldn't dance, or rather I refused to dance because I figured if I limped while walking, I would also limp while dancing. The few times I tried, I would get discouraged. Then one year I was named class president and we organized a ball. I had to attend. At the time I was dating a girl and to get some exercise we would dance in the kitchen. From then on I was less inhibited. I was twenty. I could dance to it all. When I danced to a slow song, I would use a cane but not during the jitterbug. My life changed because I felt like everyone else. I never talked about my handicap, but I could see that people were staring at me. I would say, "When they get tired of looking at me, they will look elsewhere." Often people would ask me what was wrong with me.

While I was studying at the school for fine arts, people around me said I could not make a living at painting. I switched to the Valentine Commercial Art School on Greene Avenue, and attended for one year. Afterwards I landed a job in the publicity department of Simpson's department store where I did page layouts and a little bit of drawing. Most of the illustrations were done by hand at this time. Certain artists specialized in shoes, others in fur coats or even in casseroles; I was in charge of doing last-minute corrections. I worked five years at Simpson's.

In 1949 Doug Taylor, a former president of the Quebec Society for Crippled Children, asked me to assist Miss Daigle with the summer camp. She was getting on in years. Gradually I went up the ladder, starting from assistant monitor, to monitor, and assistant director of programs, then finally director. One day Mr. Taylor said, "Instead of drawing five days a week, why don't you come to work for the handicapped and you can continue drawing on the weekend?" This was a big decision for me; I hesitated for a moment. But after a little reflection, I accepted the offer. I was director of the camp for twenty-five years, organizing fund-raising and giving conferences here and there. I really enjoyed working with the children. After Miss Daigle retired, one of her replacements, Paul Tremblay repeatedly said, "Tony, why don't you take the job of executive director of the Society? You're doing all the work. I have the salary and the title and I know nothing!" I always answered, "I'm happy in my work. We get along. I prefer to keep my job." However, when he resigned two years later, I took his place. I had the position of executive director of the Society for Crippled Children for the last twelve years of my career. I must admit this job, consisting of mostly administrative duties, did not give me as much satisfaction as my previous work with the children. The camp at St. Alphonse, which was founded in 1938, was in part my "baby". The Society sent the children to other camps until I suggested to Miss Daigle that we establish our own operation with a few tents where we could have a Scout-type camp. After visiting a piece of land at St. Alphonse, Miss Daigle made a down-payment of ten dollars that same day and we became owners of a piece of land.

It is interesting to note that at the beginning of the camp at St. Alphonse, 95 percent of the campers were polio victims.

The most difficult period of my life was the time up to age fourteen. I had to be satisfied with watching others skate and not being able to run and jump like they could. Before the founding of the Society's camp, I went to a camp with non-handicapped children and this experience was horrible. I was excluded from all the activities. I had to stand around watching others; in simple terms, I was a spectator. Each time teams were put together for a game, I was always the last one chosen. I have a firm conviction that camps today that accept handicapped children should integrate them into activities.

I got married when I was twenty-seven years old, and my wife Lucy and I have two daughters, Estelle and Noella, who are both physiotherapists.

Even though I always liked to draw and paint, the best twenty-five years of my life were those that I was director of the summer camp. I was so satisfied with my life I never thought of doing anything different.

I remember when I was young, I would take part in the annual meetings of the Society and I would meet the directors. I would tell Miss Daigle how much I liked everyone. Now that I'm retired and a board member, I sometimes remember in childhood dreaming of being on the Board of Directors.

I couldn't have had a better life. Today I find it more difficult because of fatigue and fear of going out during the winter. I have had three fractures in two years because of falls, one to my good leg and two to my polio leg. During the summer I sometimes use a wheelchair, but the snow in the winter makes it quite complicated.

About fifteen years ago, I started experiencing symptoms of post-polio syndrome. My condition has markedly deteriorated in the last eight years. At the beginning I felt more tired, I had less strength in my legs, even in my right leg that polio hadn't affected. Today there are certain movements I can't do with my good leg. I have less resistance, I tire easily, and I think my weakness continues to increase. These new weaknesses at first had me worried and I would ask myself, "When will they stop?" I often have pain, especially in my hip, and I tell my wife, "I must have bone cancer." I receive cortisone injections every two months for arthritic pain; this pain also affects my hands and my shoulders. There have been times that I was unable to get out of bed because I couldn't use my arms, my shoulders being too painful. I have a walker but I use mostly my crutches or my canes to get around; maybe if I used my walker or my wheelchair I would save my shoulders. I used to swim but I gave it up because of skin problems.

But in retrospect, I thank God for my polio because it enabled me to accomplish a job that I would never have had a chance to do otherwise. It's because of this that I consider it a privilege to have had polio.

This Way for a Reason

Jean Priest

I GOT POLIO at the age of two. When they brought me home from the hospital, I didn't even have a voice but they could tell I was crying because they could see my tears. My mother tells me I was so paralyzed that I was like a vegetable. Memories of these years, however, are inevitably coloured by what I was told by my family.

It all happened on our dairy farm in Rosemere in 1931, when I was two. I came down with a fever which the doctor diagnosed as a cold, despite the fact that there was a lot of infantile paralysis around at the time. When my two brothers, one aged three months, the other four years, also got sick, mother called the doctor back. We were all rushed to the hospital. My father often talked about how I might have contracted polio from the rubber milk bottle caps that were brought into our home before they were sterilized. In those days people would put a prepaid rubber cap into a bottle for the milkman, and my mother who did the books for the dairy farm would tally them. Only then would they be sent to the dairy for sterilization. An interesting theory. Nobody was allowed on the dairy farm for two months. The whole milking operation was closed down. We were in quarantine—the family and the milk business.

When I was brought home, Mum was thankful we had the dairy because we had access to a lot of hot water. She used to hold me in the bathtub a couple of hours a day, working my muscles and my legs. That's how I learned to swim because after a month or so I would be so relaxed she no longer had to hold me. I floated. They worked hard at getting me better. At first I had two braces right up to my hips, with locks on both sides. I remember falling. Dad was sitting in his lawn chair. I was about five. He told me, "Get up by yourself. Just pull yourself over to the fence. You can do it." I think back on all the things my parents did to force me to get moving again, one way or another. They really worked hard to get me on my feet.

My right arm never really came back. In my sixth year, they took away the brace on my right leg, and soon noticed that my ankle flapped about, so it was fused at the Children's Memorial Hospital. From then on I got around with one brace and long crutches.

One of the men who worked for my Dad was an Indian. He was a great swimmer (we lived by a river which in those days was not polluted). He went to a lot of trouble to build a beach by taking out all the rocks and putting down lots of sand from my grandfather's sandpit. So the river became easily accessible. I spent a lot of time in the water. I remember a Mrs. Gilpin, a nurse who worked at the Children's Hospital. She would come down in the afternoons and sometimes spend two hours in the water with me, swimming up and down the river. Only in later years did I realize that what she was doing was making me stronger.

When I was about fourteen it became obvious that I was developing a severe scoliosis. I was being looked after by Dr. Turner. I remember the extreme humiliation I felt when I was asked to take off my nightgown and walk with my crutches in front of a bunch of medical students and all my friends on the ward, completely naked, out on that big verandah. I just couldn't understand how he could put me through this. It was SO embarrassing. I just wanted to crawl into a hole when I got back to my bed.

I remember how I hated the cod-liver oil that we had to take every day and how we would try to throw it over the verandah into the plants if we were lucky enough to be outside when it was given to us, and the times I went flying down the big stairs at the hospital when I wasn't careful.

For my last three years of school I took a wonderful business course at the School for Crippled Children in Montreal. It was a program that was integrated into the high school program. I would take the bus from Rosemere every day into the Jean-Talon terminus where the School for Crippled Children's bus driven by that wonderful Mr. Ward—we all loved him—would pick me up at the beginning of his round. If my bus were late, he would always wait for me. My mother wasn't keen about my doing this. She thought I should stay at home and do housework. But I really wanted to take a business course. I pleaded with my father to let me try. After all, I argued, my brothers are going into town to Montreal High. So Dad went to the local minister, the Reverend Malcolm Campbell, who arranged that I be enrolled in the office training program, even though I was from out of town.

My childhood was made memorable by my family's love and protection. My two brothers watched out for my well-being. I tried doing everything they did. I tried to ski. I would fall and try again. The same with biking. My father would never say that I couldn't do it. Rather, he left the door open for me to test my limits and determine for myself what I was capable of doing. When riding a bike proved too difficult, Dad got me a horse, so I was able to keep up with my gang that way.

At age eighteen I had my hip fused because my leg came out of the socket, probably because it didn't have the requisite muscle support it needed to hold it in place. When I was about twelve Dr. Turner had insisted that I wear a huge body brace, a monstrously heavy thing made of leather with steel bars supporting it all, and laced up the front. I had to wear a cotton shirt underneath it and it would be saturated when I took it off at night. During the winter Dad would put it on the wood furnace to warm it up, which was the only comfort that contraption gave me. I'm sure it didn't do any good, but Dr. Turner contended that had I worn it as I was supposed to, my hip wouldn't have dislocated. The surgical procedure on my hip was called a Smith-Peterson pin. Nobody warned me before having this operation that it would forever be impossible to reach my feet, more especially that it would make it impossible for me to tie my shoes and I would need help with boots in the winter too. It was the shock of my life. I was in bed for eighteen months recuperating.

As I get older I realize even more what great parents I had and how intuitively well they handled the whole situation.

I found it quite difficult to get a job when I first started looking. I had to persist. Over a period of four years, I found a good job at Canadair, got married, and had a wonderful son, Glen. In 1959 I left the marriage and moved to Granby to be near my mother who could help me take care of my six-year-old Glen when I went to work. But I was doing far too much and became so run-down that I collapsed. It was difficult for the doctor to know what had happened because I was looking tanned and healthy. But he noticed that the palms of my hands were dead white. He took a blood sample. It revealed that I was dangerously anemic. So I was rushed to the hospital. It took me about a year to recover and to rebuild my stamina. Fortunately, I was living with my mother who took great care of my son while I was recovering. Glen got to love the neighbourhood, so we stayed. I eventually bought her house, and she acquired a country cottage. When she died I bought the house I now live in, and my son lives with me when he is not off doing contract work. I retired in 1989.

My post-polio symptoms began appearing in 1973. It started with my back problems at the age of forty-four. I was down at the cottage. My mother and son were away visiting my brother in PEI. One morning, all by myself, I couldn't get out of bed. I was in terrible pain. So I crawled to the telephone and told my girlfriend what had happened. She took me to the hospital in Sherbrooke. My mother had to come back to look after me. Eventually, I went to Boston for surgery, and was in intensive care for three weeks. The problems I had pulling through that surgery, including pneumonia and lungs that kept having to be drained, were attributed to my smoking. I wonder now whether it wasn't the effect of the anaesthetic. They say that some people who have polio are dangerously affected by some anaesthetics. After the operation I was positioned half standing, half sitting for six months. Why? Well, from my earlier operation, my hip wouldn't bend, and my back was straight. It was uncomfortable in the extreme. The doctor said he wanted me back for corrective hip surgery, but first I had to heal from this back operation.

I had six months leave of absence to cope with all this. They fixed me up with a special chair in the office. I kept the rest of my sick leave for the hip operation for the removal of the Smith-Peterson pin which was to be replaced with an artificial hip. There was no muscle to hold that hip, so they wired it. It was a godsend. Now I can tie my shoes. I felt like a new woman, a new wired women, for during my forties I broke my knee three times and it too is wired.

But while in Boston for a check-up in the early 1980s I remember saying to my doctor that I felt I was losing control of my body. Things were happening that I couldn't explain. He had me talk to a neurologist who had just read an article in *Time Magazine* about a new phenomenon they were calling post-polio syndrome. He said they weren't doing anything about PPS in Boston because polio was a disease of the past, but he suggested I get help back in Montreal. Later a friend watched a TV program from Toronto on which a person was being interviewed about her post-polio syndrome. She jotted down the contact number, and that is what led me to Dr. Cashman.

Dr. Cashman was a very wise man who advised me that it wouldn't be long before I would need a wheelchair. It took me two years to accept this prediction because I just couldn't imagine continuing to live in my house in the country, driving my car, and generally being independent if I was in a wheelchair. I worried about becoming house-bound.

My sister used to ask me why I didn't just get a folding wheelchair so that she could push me around the shopping centres. Then a girlfriend started persuading me in the same direction. They made it sound like so much fun. When my Mom was in the hospital in 1989 her room was far from the parking lot. The hospital corridors were long and exhausting. It was then that I decided I needed a wheelchair. I saw Dr. Cashman in June and I had my wheelchair by December. When we took it out of the back of the car my Mom started to cry, thinking of how hard they had worked to get me strong enough to get around without this kind of help. It was very difficult for her. There's a man in Granby who maintains it, but I have to go to the Constance Lethbridge in Montreal to get the cushions positioned properly. It is comfortable and supports me beautifully.

The medications I'm on now are Mestinon (it's not without side effects for me) and something for my osteoarthritis. But the major problem I have had to deal with, and may it be the last, are the bits of metal in my spine from the surgery I had in the 1970s. They were breaking off, causing sores and infections. For over two years I tried to get the problem resolved. It's a real saga of lost records, unanswered messages, and a frustrating lack of coordination. My phone bills to the Royal Vic alone were over $100. A doctor I consulted in Boston said the metal, if removed, would have to be replaced by Harrington rods, which would have been a serious undertaking. By 1998 my back problem became so severe that I had to be rushed to the Royal Victoria Hospital where Dr. Abie did an emergency procedure. They CAT-scanned my spine and found where the infection had built up around my spine. I was there for two and a half weeks. With the help of the CLSC, I was able to come home attached, from November to March, to an intravenous of antibiotics. Thank heaven for my son Glen who would pick up the raw materials from the drugstore and take them to the pharmacy at the hospital in Granby to be made up into solutions. When they were ready, they would call him to pick them up and store them in the fridge. The CLSC would then come and change my IV bags. When finally the tube fell out of its own accord, undoubtedly from having been in too long, I went to the hospital and they replaced the IV treatment with pills. From this experience I became acutely aware of the inefficiencies of Quebec's healthcare system, but appreciative of its ultimate effectiveness because now that this episode is all over, I feel I have been well cared for. My balance combined with my increased weakness require me to rely completely on my wheelchair now, so I am planning to have my kitchen adapted.

Polio certainly has affected my life. Perhaps I would have been a pilot if I hadn't had polio; when I tried for my pilot's license, it was denied. I subsequently enjoyed soaring and sailing. Polio has taught me tolerance and acceptance. I firmly believe that God made me this way for a reason. I'm very happy within myself.

Adjust, but Keep Going

Reverend William (Bill) Phillips

Nightmares! I knew I was yelling. It was 1934. Although then but four and a half years old, memories of that night sixty-five years ago remain etched in my mind as if it was yesterday. I felt I was falling and was screaming for someone to catch me. Although my parents and the family doctor, Dr. Farris, stood around the bed, it seemed to me they were like statues, paralyzed and unable to reach out.

At the hospital the doctor talked of double pneumonia. The next day I was sent from the Brantford hospital to Hamilton. My dad's boss offered the use of his car. En route I felt very sick. My vomiting in the boss's luxury coupe was not really in Dad's plans. We stopped the car and a lady dressed in white came out of a big house carrying a glass of water. She seemed to me to be like an angel. I remember little after that except that they diagnosed the problem as infantile paralysis (polio) and explained that my father had to stay away from the house for a short time because a sign saying "Quarantine–Polio" was to be placed on our front door.

The following three months in the Brantford General Hospital are but a blur to me now. I remember being strapped down to a metal frame. They told my parents that they must immobilize my legs to make the pain stop. My dad was not ready to accept the thought of having a handicapped child unable to walk so he acted on the advice of the family chiropractor Dr. Clark, and had me removed from the hospital.

Dr. Clark assured Dad that in exercising my limbs he would have me walking within a year. Every day except Sundays, I was carried to Dr. Clark's office for a treatment. My mother, helped by a friend, would carry me into the back yard, place me so that my legs were in direct sunlight and then spend hours moving my legs back and forth. I have but scant memories of those days.

Nine months after leaving the hospital, by leaning on others I was able to stand for short periods and place some weight on my legs. Dr. Clark made a house call and persuaded my parents it was time for me to begin to walk. This scene I remember very clearly. They helped me out of the bedroom, adjacent to the kitchen, and had me lean on the edge of the wood stove. I took a few steps, holding onto the stove. They then said "Now walk on your own to the table." It was probably only about four steps away, but I made it! What a day!

At this time my father's pride was sorely wounded by ill health, unemployment, the backlash of the Great Depression, being on welfare, and coping with a handicapped child. His mother had died when he was very young and from age thirteen on he had been on his own. He had worked on the Great Lakes freighters, then after marriage, on the fish tugs in Port Dover, Ontario. He prided himself in being self-sufficient. But now his world seemed to have crashed in around him. Not knowing where to turn he began to listen to the friends who had helped with my polio and who had offered encouragement during those difficult times. Most were involved in an evangelical church located just across from our home. One day, Dad agreed to attend their church. The gospel message gripped his heart, changing his life and the entire direction of our home. My most vivid memory of church services, however, was enviously watching the other kids slide down the banister after church. An usher, reading my mind, looked around to make sure my Dad wasn't watching, lifted me up and let me slide down too. The sermons didn't stick, but the usher's interest in and understanding of a five-and-a-half-year-old, did. Now I could be like others.

By fall we had moved into a different house located just one block from a school. Each day a neighbour boy pulled me to school in my wagon. With continued physiotherapy by my parents and their friends plus continued treatment by Dr. Clark with his insistence on aquatic and tricycle exercises, strength was regained and walking, even running became a possibility. Recollections of my childhood from that point on are very positive. Although I could not enter all sports, life seemed to me to be quite normal. In baseball, I would hit the ball, but a friend would run for me. In fact, my sister, two years older than I, has no recollection of my being "a cripple". Actually, I never recall my parents talking about my polio nor do I remember ever having complained about having had polio. By the age of twelve I was delivering groceries after school using my bicycle. Most customers were unaware of my weakness. For me, as with many other polio survivors, life had become a challenge. If I couldn't peddle up a hill like other kids, I'd simply return later and keep trying until I could. I enjoyed music and played the violin in the High School orchestra. I became very involved in activities at the church. Never do I remember feeling that my childhood polio had put a damper on things.

From the age of ten I wanted to do missionary service. This led me to becoming a Baptist minister. Although I had wanted to work in Africa, I was encouraged instead to look at our own country as a mission field. My first parish was Ville Émard in Montreal during which time I married Blanche

Ford. We had four children.

I had been told that once you got over polio, its effects were finished. While working in Sept-Îles, the cold winters of Quebec's North Shore area brought on repeated problems of bronchial pneumonia. After six years of ministry there, my diminished health forced us to leave and return to Montreal. Important therapy for me, and perhaps it can be attributed to my having polio, was to set ambitious goals and see those goals attained. Despite my health I was fortunate in being able to achieve the planting of fifty-two French-speaking Baptist churches in Quebec.

The times of weakness, fatigue, and pain first experienced in Sept-Îles worsened. For no apparent reason I would fall. I noticed when kicking a football with the grandchildren that my "good leg" would let me down. For over six years I went from doctor to doctor, specialist to specialist, hospital to hospital trying to find the answer to my decreasing mobility, increased pain and increased weakness. Following every examination I would be told, "We thought it was multiple sclerosis but it does not completely check out as that. We have found nothing wrong with you." This answer brought little comfort while sprawled out on the lawn or sidewalk or at the bottom of a flight of stairs. At one point I was referred to a physiotherapist, but after a few sessions the therapist realized that the more I exercised, the worse things became. She suggested I stop.

My wife and I wondered if a career change might help. I had been driving between eighty and one hundred thousand miles per year crisscrossing Quebec and Canada in the interests of our Quebec ministry. A normal work week would often reach sixty to eighty hours. Thus in 1990 we returned to our first love, ministry in a local parish, and we became involved in the development of a new church in the West Island area of Montreal.

Two pastor friends, one in Toronto, the other in Victoria, British Columbia, had polio symptoms similar to mine. My friend in British Columbia said he had been diagnosed with post-polio syndrome. While at times I had wondered if my problems were polio-related, I relied on information given by most sources that polio left only the limitations received at the time of contracting the disease. I was surprised when he told me the best post-polio clinic in the country was in Montreal! I wasted no time in contacting Dr. Neil Cashman, director of the Polio Clinic at the Montreal Neurological Institute and Hospital.

It may seem strange but for me it was good news to know I had the post-polio syndrome. As someone has said, "Better the devil you know than the devil you do not know." I had some calculated decisions to make. I now knew strength and mobility would continue to decrease. We set a retirement date. We moved into a house that could be adapted for a wheelchair. Although I had graduated from one cane to two, soon I would need Canadian crutches, then a manual wheel chair. When we renovated our back deck we added a ramp and included another ramp in the front landscaping plans. An elevator in the bathtub allows me to get into a hot bath when pain becomes too intense. An occupational therapist helped us rethink the layout of our home office. More recently, with decreased use of my shoulders and arms, I have become eligible for help with the expenses of a motorized wheelchair and an adapted van. Grab bars, different-styled door hinges, replacement taps, remodeling of the steps from the garage to the kitchen—all have been undertaken with a view to insuring continued independent movement and mobility. It has been a little more difficult to control my agenda. Accepting only one major activity a day and scheduling for an after-dinner rest period remain challenges.

The fact of having a very supportive wife, children, and grandchildren, an interesting hobby (woodworking), many loyal friends, and involvement in church and community projects all add up to a joie de vivre that adds anticipation to each new day. My last word to fellow polios: "Don't dread the changes. Anticipate them and prepare for them; adjust and keep going and don't lose faith."

Never Give Up

CHARLIE BROCKLEHURST

MY BODY NEVER DEVELOPED like my brother's and sister's because of the effect polio had on me. It struck in 1934. I was six years old. We lived in Montreal. I was never very strong, in fact, a delicate child. But I'm a survivor—a fighter. I think that's from my mother's side of the family. She instilled into me the notion that if you have something wrong with you, you fight it. You don't wallow in self-pity feeling sorry for yourself. She would never let me do that when I was small. I guess it was very hard on her when I got sick. Most mothers would naturally want to baby you, protect you and tell you that everything was going to be all right. But not my mother.

One Sunday, when she returned from church, she noticed me walking down the hall in a peculiar way, holding onto the walls, unable to walk straight. She chastised me for imitating a drunken man. "It's not nice," she said. I replied that it was the way I walked. Once again she told me to stop it. In those days you did what you were told. My parents were firm with us. Punishment consisted of having pocket money withheld, that kind of thing; we weren't beaten. So my mother picked me up and called my father saying, "There's something wrong with him. All his bones are as if they are cracking. I think the child has polio." I can still hear my father's words. "You've been reading about polio. It must be in your brain. Just because Johnny next door has polio, you think Charlie has it too." But from the way I was walking, there was no question something was wrong. My mother then called Westmount's Dr. Ashton Kerr. His advice was to get me to the hospital quickly.

I was rushed into a cab, taken to the Children's Memorial Hospital, and left there. I was frightened. Everything was so different. Everyone was grabbing me. All I could do was cry. Doctors were sticking needles into me and I had no idea what was happening. Then I heard that I would have to stay in the hospital and my parents would have to leave. I worked myself into a nervous wreck. Although I was only there for about three months, it seemed like a lifetime. I wasn't allowed to see my parents for fear I would get too emotional, wanting to go home. But they visited the hospital every day and were able to see me through a one-way window. I could hear their voices and would get all excited. I was taunted into getting better by the promise of being able to see my parents only when I recovered, and not until then. Nonetheless I was sent a parcel almost every second day with a toy or candy. My father worked at the bank where there were about 100 employees, and many of them gave my father toys to bring to me, so I ended up with a lot of very nice playthings.

There were two of us in a room. I played with all these toys either on the floor, on a blanket, or in my bed. I would be taken almost every day to The Tank. They would strap me to a board, slide me into the warm water and try to work my arm and my leg. It was painful; in fact to me it was torture. And I would yell, "It hurts! It hurts!" But they would calmly just tell me to move this, move that. I thought it was stupid. I would be returned to my room absolutely exhausted. After three months I was sort of walking, dragging my leg behind me. I couldn't stand on it because it was too weak. They fitted me with a brace to hold me up. My left leg was just too weak. My mother objected to my dependency upon this support. However I needed it for a few years. Was I glad when I could wear long pants which covered this contraption on my leg! I could look more like the other boys. It was then that the doctor suggested I stop using the brace. So one Saturday night when I was getting ready to go out with my parents—being the youngest, they took me everywhere with them—I couldn't find my brace. My mother, who was a meticulous house-keeper, had trained us to put everything where it belonged. But my brace was nowhere. My mother said, "I'm tired of telling you people that when you take off a thing you put it in the right place so you can find it. We're late now. We've got no time to be fooling around looking for a brace, so go without it." I was sputteringly mad, being blamed for something I had nothing to do with. But having got me mad, I was able to do the impossible. Before I knew it I was in the car without my brace. "You see," said my father, "you are managing perfectly well without your brace. I don't know what you are sputtering about."

On Sunday I was made to go to Church without the brace. And on Monday, there was school. What was I going to do, because the brace was apparently still nowhere to be found? My father asserted that although he worked for the bank, he didn't own it and was in no position to buy another brace if I was so careless with the one I had. I knew that my brace couldn't have disappeared, but my parents were determined that I wasn't going to get it back. My father told me to get on with it. I was to walk to school, and if I got tired I could sit on someone's steps to rest. So when I returned home from school, my father asked me how many times I had sat on someone's steps. Well, of course, I hadn't needed to rest. Then they asked me if I wanted to be fitted for a new brace, at which point I was the one who said I didn't need one. Then my mother told me what had happened to that old brace. She had put it into the furnace. And that was the end of braces for me.

To keep me moving my family always got me to answer the phone, and to answer the doorbell. I objected, saying, "I'm like a little bellboy around here." The phone was never for me. Running was what they wanted me to do, and this was as good a way as any to strengthen my leg. Being annoyed had me rushing all the time. My mother felt this was a sign of determination. These tricks were their way of getting me strong.

As for my face, it was all twisted. I remember when my parents carried me down the big staircase at the Children's Memorial Hospital on my way home, I heard my mother say to the doctor, "That child's face!" The doctor exhorted her to remember that I was young and that maybe the serum would work. "We think it is working because he isn't paralyzed as badly as many others." This serum had been flown in from New York for me. My mother with determination declared that if she did nothing else, she was going to get my face back to normal. We had to keep the muscles alive and get them strong again.

So every day she took me on the streetcar and up that big hill to the hospital. I would have to take time off from school to go to the hospital. Every night I would have a hot bath, soak in it and work my leg, and, with oil, my father would rub my arm, rub my leg, put it up, put it down, work on my face. I resisted every moment of it. I was really terrible. My mother was the therapist and she bore the brunt of my discontent. But it worked. Only when I get tired now does my face show signs of the old polio. It will twitch. Recently I had bypass surgery. Doctors noticed my affected face and asked whether I had had a stroke.

When I was twenty-one Dr. Kerr told me, "If anything goes wrong with your head—if you find any unusual pain, something in your ears—go to a doctor or to a hospital right away." I confided to my Mother after my hospital experience that never would I go to a doctor, a nurse, or a hospital in all my life. I hated them all.

I remember once when I was still in school, we were at the airport going to Vancouver and I got a pain in the middle of my stomach. I thought it was an ulcer, probably from nerves and fear from trying to cope with school and all the children, trying to be like them when I couldn't be. Because I was different they just wrote me off as being unable to join in. I didn't have the strength to run or to throw when it came to sports like baseball, hockey, or skating. I felt left out. Even though my father and two brothers were good sportsmen, I was told that it would be useless to try these sports myself because I wouldn't be able to do them. So when my father took my brothers to hockey games, I was not included. Instead my parents planned something special like visits to the museum. They always gave me a treat to make up for what I couldn't do.

Going away to see the musical *South Pacific* was the first thing I had ever asked for, and after a lot of soul-searching my parents gave me the train ticket, the hotel, and a ticket to the show, making me promise to phone home every night to reassure them I was alright.

When I was younger, I adored my toys, my electric trains. I had a whole basement full of things to do. Sometimes young friends would join me, but if they didn't come, I wasn't bothered. I could amuse myself. I enjoyed my own company. I'm never bored, never lonesome. I like watching good movies and listening to the opera. The atmosphere in a room is important to me.

I live up to my sun sign, which is Leo, liking the theatre and the make-believe world. I travel quite a bit and love sightseeing. But I'll never go to beaches or to a swimming pool after my experience in "the tank" in the hospital. A pool to me means therapy and hospital. Despite numerous invitations to go to Florida and other seaside places, I just will not go. It would be a waste of time and money. If I go in water over my knees, I have to get out in a hurry. I can still feel that sensation of being on the board. I only take showers—never a bath!

I'm quite different from my brothers and sisters. More like my mother. She was artistic, and had a good eye for fashion. Having a nice home and entertaining well were important to her as they are to me. I guess it's in my genes.

Teachers were kind, but I was left on my own a lot. At recess time I would just go and read. It was the same at home. I would never go out to play with the neighbourhood kids. My family was tuned into this behaviour and would console me by saying hockey wasn't all that much fun anyway. I would sit on the floor and cry sometimes, and my mother would come along and pull me out of my depression by reminding me of all the things I could do. Her therapy included having me sit on the floor and she would put a sock on my foot and tie a rag to my good leg pretending she was tired and needed help polishing floors, pretending also to forget that it was the strong leg she was preparing for floor polishing. Before long I would suggest alternating the legs, so that way I got some good exercise, and I enjoyed it. She would play tricks on me all the time. Because I was tall, she would ask for my help in dusting those hard-to-reach places. "I'm getting old," she would say, "and can't reach," even though she was only forty and as spry as could be. But I was home and helped her. She kept me going all the time, and that was therapy too, without my knowing it.

The doctors were aware of her dedication, saying she would never give up on me. She even had me chewing gum for my jaw muscles. When I got tired of the gum, she would give me toffee. That was delicious exercise! You can just picture how I had to work my mouth full of that sticky stuff. Dr. Kerr used to tell me that I should be very grateful that I had a mother that was so good to me.

I was always interested in music and the arts, theatre and opera. When I went for a walk, I would look at store windows and marvel at their beauty. It would draw me into the stores. When I was old enough I would take the streetcar and wander around looking at the decorations or go to museums to pass my time. All this influenced my career choice, which was interior decorating.

There wasn't insurance in those days, but we were comfortably off. My father worked for the bank. I remember my mother saying during the Depression that those who have must help those who are not so fortunate. She would help people on relief, making food for their large families, or buying cotton to make sheets for them. "It's good to help people," she would say. My father paid for everything. Perhaps they had to do without certain things, but I didn't feel it. It's only now that I'm older I realize that they probably had to sacrifice things like travel to pay for doctors' and hospital bills.

There was seventeen years' difference in age between me and my oldest brother. He would take me to his place on occasional weekends to give my family a break. My parents would never leave me alone for fear that there might be a fire, that I would panic and be unable to get out. Even though my brother's place was only about twenty blocks from home. It was a real treat for me to get away. We would go for walks or go to one of Moira Shearer's Saturday morning shows.

As a family we would go to the country in the summer. This clean fresh air was "good for Charles's health. It will build him up," my parents would say. This made me hate the country just as I hated water. We were about a mile and a half from the village so I had to walk to get the mail. My father would come for the weekends, and often times, a lot of visitors too. When I was sixteen I said to my mother that I refused to go to the country ever again. The sky is just as blue in town, and that is where I wanted to be. I'd rather go downtown to Peel and Ste. Catherine Street, look at the store windows, go to the Museum. That was better than being buried alive in the country just looking at trees waving in the wind and the grass growing. That was my opinion of the country. The Town of Mount Royal and Westmount were country enough for me! I've lived in Montreal all my life.

Polio affected what I really wanted to be in life. Had it not been for my health, I think I would have been a priest. This was a calling from early childhood. I became very depressed when my doctor advised my parents that such a vocation would be too taxing on what he thought was a fragile body. Being an obedient and trusting person, I accepted this advice, knowing that it must be for my own good. I wasn't able to share this profound disappointment with my friends because I even feared their sympathy.

I got ulcers that summer from keeping everything locked in, being unable to do that which was most important to me, just as I had been restricted as a young man. I remember coming down the elevator in the Medical Arts Building having seen yet another doctor. He told me I would have to be hospitalized because I had an ulcer. I couldn't bear it. When I was waiting for the streetcar on the corner of Guy and Sherbrooke I saw a big cement truck coming down Côte-des-Neiges. So I stepped off the curb, hoping to end my life. I'd had enough disappointments. But a kind couple screamed at me and pulled me back. They found a doctor's appointment card in my pocket, so they took me back to the doctor's office I had just left. I was in hysterics, falling to pieces. I'll never forget this couple. Their name was Macdonald. They drove me home and when I told them that I was nothing but trouble for my parents, they said "Parents don't think that way," and they convinced me that life wasn't really all that bad. I was admitted to the hospital the next day. The treatment for my ulcers was buttermilk and raw oysters, no operation. I haven't touched an oyster since. I still have the ulcers, but I took care of them by eating lots of cream, custards, and the like. I was told never to get a taste for liquor or spices or heavy seasonings. So I learned at a young age to be careful about my diet.

My whole life has been doctors, hospitals, clinics. I thought when I got older I would have a break. I was lucky to have a mother who kept repeating, "You can master this ... you can master that." But now it's my heart. In the mid- 1990s I was on my way out West when at the airport I got a horrible pain at the very moment I was taking out travel insurance. I was putting the forms I had filled out into the mailbox when I realized that I couldn't travel feeling the way I was. I grabbed my luggage before it was put on the plane, got into a cab, and returned home. Luckily my doctor was able to see me right away, so I walked the three blocks to his office. The nurse was shocked at my appearance and got me into the doctor's office immediately. Within seconds he was asking his nurse to call 911 while telling me, "You have had either a massive heart attack or you are going to have one." I almost fell off the table. I was taken to Intensive Care at St. Mary's Hospital, and then within three weeks, to the Royal Victoria Hospital for tests and observation and finally by-pass surgery. Dr. Latimer was my surgeon. He reassured me that given my perfect condition, the risk factor was between three and five percent, and that I should have the operation and enjoy another good twenty years. Without the surgery he believed my life expectancy would be less than a year.

In preparing me for the operation a nurse who was about to give me a sedating needle commented on how calm I was. She said it was unusual that a patient undergoing what I was about to could sleep all night without the help of sleeping pills. He said that most patients are terrified to be left alone. I answered him by saying that I've gotten used to it in life. I had thought that all my problems would be over when I grew up, but now I realize that nothing is ever going to be right with me. It's just one thing after another. But I guess polio was the worst because it prevented me from doing what I really wanted to do. Whatever happens, I've learned to go along with it.

I got Ménière's syndrome about forty years ago, just after getting ulcers. I had the two types of dizziness. If I got an attack it would throw me right off a chair. I was in the kitchen about four years ago taking a pill by the sink, and the force of it threw me back till I smashed into the refrigerator. I had to have bars put up in the bathroom so that I could hold on in case I were to have an attack while in the shower. The best thing was to sit on the floor if an attack came on. An attack could last from an hour to five hours. If I were in bed I would have to crawl to the bathroom and keep my head over the toilet bowl where I would vomit up yellowish bile coming apparently from my ears. Prior to my heart surgery, I had quite a few dreadful attacks, but I haven't had one since just after that surgery.

With my heart problem I'm on a low-fat diet. It means going to a team of doctors to be followed up every six months.

I'm not married, at first because I thought I might have a religious vocation, and later when that was ruled out, because I didn't see how I could support anyone but myself with all the health problems I was having. Looking back I'm relieved that I didn't have any dependents. I've always been very active in groups and societies, and in my work I help people and keep very busy. Being on a committee for the restoration of a heritage building has been particularly rewarding.

My life hasn't been what I wanted it to be, but that happens to a lot of people. I don't feel sorry for myself and I'm no longer worried about dying. I'm going to continue and take things as they come. I've told my family that should they get a phone call, or should a policeman come to the door telling them I had dropped dead on the street, they are to know that that is how I wanted it to be. I must admit I'm scared of having a stroke paralyze me. I want to live my life fully until the very end. That's my mother's influence telling me to keep going.

Even though my brothers and sisters are older than I, they have always come to me for advice. "Why?" I would ask my mother, "why do they come to me when I am the youngest? I should be going to them." She replied, "You are more mature, more sensible. Sickness does that. It takes a lot out of you." Two days before she died she called me in and said, "I'm not going to get over this.

When I'm gone, take care of yourself. Look at all the family in the next room. They can't cope with sickness and death. Who's the strong one now? Who's leaning on you now? I am." She told me that all her bills were paid, and her will was going to treat all four children alike, except for her pin money which she wanted me to use for a trip to California, the trip I hadn't been able to take because I didn't want to be away should my mother need me. She probably told the rest of the family to look out for me because they were all right by me when I had that heart surgery.

I have had no trouble with my old polio and only think of it if I see a movie with a polio victim in it. Then I am reminded of how lucky I have been.

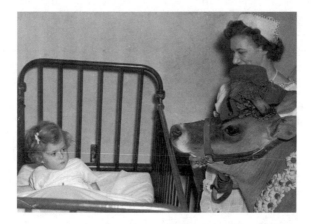

A polio patient receives a visit from Elsie the Borden cow.
Courtesy of Polio Canada

Keep Going the Full Mile

Dr. Herta Guttman

One of the legacies of polio is that I do not like the feeling of being powerless, reminiscent of when I was unable to move from the waist down. I found it humiliating not to be able to keep up physically with other kids who had never had to cope with impairment. It's only in recent years that I realize that there is a downside to that. I wasn't pushed to get up and moving until six months after the initial polio, which was the passive Sister Kenny method. Nor was I supposed to go up or down stairs, so I went down on my bottom. I had to miss school for a year.

Doctors were uncertain that my second bout was polio because at that time they doubted that it could recur. Both times polio affected my legs. This was very clear from the kind of exhaustion I experienced from my day's activity back then, such as helping my mother redo the gravel driveway. All the neighbourhood children were spreading the gravel, pulling full pails up to the rooftop porch above the garage. Towards the evening, I could hardly walk. My doctor consulted an orthopedist and I remember him saying, "Come to me, come to me." He obviously thought I had hysterical paralysis. I remember trying to walk towards him, feeling absolutely horrible because I knew I was going to fall. I did. And then I was taken to the Neuro for the second time. Wonderful Dr. Donald E. McEachern was my doctor. He was so humane—a lovely man. I only found out many years later that it was exceptional for young children to be patients of the Neuro. I also learned that his good words on my behalf helped me to get into St. George's School.

From my time at the Neuro I particularly remember sitting in one of the covered porches with my mother. It was like a room. (I think they are all gone now.) The view was spectacular. With us was a boy with a plaster cast on his head. He couldn't read. I was reading books such as the Mary Jane series that described adventures in many different countries. I thought I was so lucky. It's probably the reason I developed a strong interest in traveling.

My memories are confused between my two bouts with polio. My first memory of getting polio was when I fell off a ledge from a window onto a balcony. Throughout my school years there were certain things I couldn't do in gym. I always lagged behind when a bunch of kids were running. Nor was I good at things like rope climbing.

My mother insisted upon staying with me in the hospital, which was absolutely against all rules. She created such a scene—she being a very strong-willed woman, they caved in and converted a treatment room to accommodate us. I also remember my father visiting me and bringing me goldfish. Dr. Penfield came to visit me, probably because he was interested in the fact I had the symptoms of polio and had contracted the disease twice. I also remember being injected with vitamins twice a day.

I really thought little of my polio until a few years ago. To all intents and purposes, I had recovered, except when I was skating or running, or things like that. Because I didn't look handicapped I was able to deny to myself that perhaps I never really had polio. I was very hard on myself for being unable to do everything that others were doing. I remember so distinctly when I was at school two boys were talking about me, and not necessarily behind my back, saying, "She could play baseball if she wanted. She's tall and she could do it, but she just doesn't want to." Of course, I knew I couldn't.

I only found out why years later when I went to the Polio Clinic at West Park Hospital in Toronto and read a lot of articles given to me by the social worker about the psychological aspects of polio. It was through these articles that I discovered that it's quite usual for ex-polio children to be amongst the most motivated, highly striving of all the disabled, and the most successful. I think a lot of it has to do with the way we were exhorted to "keep up": "You must exercise," "You must this, and you must that."

I don't think I was in the hospital for more than two or three weeks. Whether I could or couldn't walk was irrelevant because I wasn't allowed to walk for six months. I had to rest at home. My parents would carry me onto the porch in the morning and back. My treatment consisted of massage and passive exercises twice a week, and exercises in the pool at the Children's Memorial up on the hill. I hated physiotherapy and massages and still avoid them, doubtless because of my earlier experiences.

It wasn't easy on my mother. She and my father had come from Austria in 1930. She spoke English, but not at all well. She did speak French though. She fought "them" on my behalf tooth and nail at the Neuro, in spite of their prejudices and rules. Looking back, it was perhaps a bad thing for my sister that my mother left the home to be with me. My sister was only eight months old at the time—just the time of life when children have a lot of separation anxiety. My grandmother stayed with her and thereafter she seemed to be closer to her than to my mother. I think I could have managed at least overnight without her, but her anxiety for me kept her nearby.[1]

I married in 1953 and had two daughters, and in spite of my weak abdominal muscles, I gave birth without an anesthetic. When I was about fifty I started stumbling, tripping over cracks in the pavement, things like that, so I went to see an orthopedist, Dr. Sullivan at St. Mary's Hospital. He had been in Hong Kong and seen a lot of post-polio patents. When I told him I had had polio, he was quick to diagnose me as having post-polio syndrome. That was in 1984. I'd never heard of it before, so he explained it to me. I went to see Dr. Cashman at the Montreal Neurological Institute, but he didn't yet have a polio team. Then I heard there was a Post-Polio Clinic at West Park Hospital in Toronto.[2]

For the greater part of my life, polio hadn't really bothered me, although looking back I remember that I would always tire easily. I was always pushing myself, and often I would have leg cramps in the middle of the night, but it didn't stop me. I even wore high heels on that hilly McGill campus. I don't get those cramps now, but I get very, very tired, so I have a rest every day and pace myself. For instance, if I am going to be on my feet a lot, I do without my morning walk on the mountain that day. But I managed to keep up with my work in medical school, even giving birth to our first daughter during my studies. We now have two daughters—one in Toronto, the other in Utica. They both have children, so life goes on.

On the whole people aren't aware that I had polio. They sometimes notice the tremor in my hands. But until I had a consultation with Dr. Trojan, I believed that this was a familial trait, unaware that polio could affect the upper body. Dr. Trojan set me right. Polio can affect the whole body. My little granddaughter notices the tremor all the time, but my own children never noticed it, from which I deduce that it must be more apparent (worse) now. It never stopped me from doing anything, though. My thigh muscles sometimes get cramps—probably because they are most used when standing, cooking, things like that.

I wish I could have been more athletic. Although I did cross-country ski, I was never very good at it. Now, just to get my skis on is a whole production, what with my drop toe. To put on the new kind of gear you have to lift your toe. For a long time I have been stumbling over that dropped toe. Dr. Trojan feels I don't need a brace to correct this problem. After all, it's a dropped toe, not a dropped foot. But I wonder. I would love to be able to accompany my husband skiing. He's a great alpine skier. He also loves sailing. I would like to feel less clumsy when on the boat with him.

Because of what I know of the achievements of people who have had polio, I'm quite proud that I'm part of that group that has succeeded so well in life. We probably have something to say to people with other disabilities in terms of how you manage your disability and live a normal life. What struck me when I had my first appointment at West Park was a young Asian woman who was using a brace and a cane, which made my problem seem trivial, i.e., I couldn't go cross-country skiing. At West Park they were taken aback by this complaint at first, but everything is a question of degree. I wasn't measuring up to my husband's ability either in strength or stamina and I wanted to know why. Now that I know and my husband understands, he's always after me to sit down. Anything to avoid cramps at night. I don't look as if I need to be so careful; it's a problem. I remember many years ago as a young married woman these cramps would wake me up out of my sleep. My husband was terrified. I had never mentioned this problem to him. At that time I didn't realize it had anything to do with my old polio.

Someone who was very special to me as an example was Franklin Delano Roosevelt. I remember wanting a Scottie dog like his but my parents wouldn't hear of it.

Nonetheless, polio has been an asset to my life. Even though it might be a chicken and egg dilemma, I believe my medical sensitivity has been enriched through this experience with polio and that, who knows, perhaps that is why I entered the field of medicine. I understand how people feel when they are ill and I have learned over the years that we know our bodies best. How can you tell someone they aren't experiencing something they are experiencing?

I am just beginning to experience the consequences of having had polio as a child. I am trying to listen to the cautionary messages my overused muscles are giving me as I push myself to the limit in a stressful job as a psychiatrist and until recently, director of Montreal's prestigious Allan Memorial Institute.

My greatest hope is that present research on the post-polio syndrome may lead to better understanding of other neurological diseases in which degeneration of the nerve cells is a prominent feature. My motto: "They also serve who only stand and wait."

Countless Repetitions, and It Worked

Elizabeth (Treglown) Goodfellow

I GOT POLIO while my family was on vacation in North Hatley, Quebec, early in September 1942 at the age of seventeen. The doctor there was in his eighties and had never seen a case. It started with the flu, then stiffness in my neck. When I awoke in the middle of the night with a temperature of 104 and was having difficulty breathing, I was sent into Montreal by ambulance accompanied by my mother. It was very hot. The ambulance driver took us to the Royal Victoria Hospital, not knowing where the Montreal Neurological Institute and Hospital was. When the admitting nurse realized why I was there she said with some alarm, "This is the maternity hospital! Take her to the Neuro."

The admitting doctor at the Neuro was Dr. Herbert Modlin. He told my mother I had either polio or spinal meningitis. She promptly dropped a bottle of Old Spice cologne. It broke and the whole place smelled. Dr. Modlin asked her which doctor she wanted. She had no idea as we had only lived in Montreal two years so he suggested Dr. Francis McNaughton. There were only two of us polios in the Neuro, me and Ken Hugessen.

My fever was high and I had been filled with barbiturates to knock me out. Dr. Francis McNaughton called in Dr. Struthers who had recently sent a nurse to Minneapolis, Minnesota to learn the Sister Kenny treatment. She had just returned and Dr. Struthers was anxious to try this method on me. He warned my parents that it would be very expensive. I would need two nurses on each shift. At the beginning the treatment consisted of hot packs changed every twenty minutes by day and every two hours at night. The packs were made from old wool blankets cut into small pieces. Each piece was put in a tub of hot or boiling water and put through a wringer in order for it to be as dry as possible. The packs were put on my affected parts and covered with pieces of rubber sheeting to retain the heat. They had to pull me in and out of the iron lung for this treatment. Within ten days my breathing started to come back so they were able to start physiotherapy. I'm absolutely convinced that I owe my recovery to the diligence and intensive care of those young nurses.

I was completely paralyzed on my left side to my waist. I had some movement in my right arm but I couldn't straighten my legs. The packs alleviated the spasm. When it was decided I was breathing properly, they took me out of the iron lung. Suddenly I started having difficulty. My wonderful Nurse Collett rushed to get the intern. I remember not being able to breathe and feeling as if I were going backwards. I had one of those dreams where I saw my whole life—it was all dark green with flashes of things I had done. And there was a light at the end of the tunnel. I didn't find it peaceful. I remember very distinctly knowing I was dying and said to myself, "I don't want to die and I'm not going to." When I came to there was a big suction tube down my throat and a whole bunch of doctors around me. Dr. Struthers was there, and when they pulled out the tube, I said very vehemently, "I don't want to die." He assured me that I wouldn't. All the barbiturates they had given me had depressed my breathing. Dr. Rasmussen was chief intern and ordered me off this medication immediately. It was also making me hallucinate and causing unusual sleepiness. The nurses would tell the doctors about this, but when they asked me, "How are you?" I would come to and say, "Fine!" So it took a while before they took my hallucinations and drowsiness seriously.

Ken Hugessen wasn't so lucky. His total paralysis confined him to bed and the iron lung. His father wrote of him: "It needs little imagination to picture what it must have been like, for a boy who was accustomed to an active existence and was a lover of the outdoor life, to be motionless in a hospital room for weeks on end, unable to move hand or foot and dependent on others for the simplest of needs." He told his parents that he had never known a dull moment in the hospital. I would go and visit Ken in my wheelchair, even though by then I could walk. I didn't want him to be discouraged by my recovery. He started to get stronger, but never got over the weakening effects of a flu. Just before Christmas he died in his sleep, leaving an inspired collection of his poetry as a memorial.[1]

After about a month and a half at the Neuro, I was transferred to the Ross Pavilion. I don't think the supervisor at the Ross wanted me, probably because it would be difficult to find a place to set up the washing machines and the hot water tubs for hot pack treatment. But they needed my room at the Neuro for someone else. Because of this transfer, my hot pack treatment lapsed for two days. When Dr. Struthers found out, all hell broke loose.

Dr. Struthers was a real taskmaster. The nurses seemed terrified of him. When I was in the iron lung, the nurses would paint my nails bright red. I developed a rash around my eyes and around my mouth. The nurses pointed this out to Dr. Struthers, asking what he thought could have caused it, and without a moments hesitation he uttered, "That filthy nail polish. Get rid of it." Amazingly enough, the rash went when the polish was removed. I haven't been able to wear nail polish since.

The nurses used to come in and tell me about the seasick machine in the Neuro. They were bringing in sailors, putting them in the seasick machine and giving them pills like Dramamine to see if this would stop them throwing up at sea. Many years later I mentioned this to Head Nurse Flanagan. She looked horrified because this research was supposed to have been wartime "top secret."

I remember those months vividly and thinking how terrible it must have been for my parents. We had come from England in 1940, during the war. Our lives had already been disrupted, and to have this happen was the crowning blow. But life went on. My sister Ann married when I was in the Neuro, and she and Charles came up to the Neuro right after their wedding.

When Sister Kenny came to Montreal, Dr. Struthers invited me to meet her at the Children's Memorial Hospital.

A very sad incident was Nurse Buchanan's suicide. My mother was devastated. This nurse had done so much to make me better, and we would have done anything to help her had we known in time of her distress.

By the fall of 1943 I was virtually better, so I accompanied my sister to Washington where there was a major outbreak of polio. My sister-in-law had a friend who wrote a column for one of the papers sponsoring Sister Kenny to set up her treatment program in a Washington hospital. Because physicians were skeptical of the Sister Kenny treatment, there was a lot of opposition to her from polio people in the States. When my sister-in-law told them about me, and that I had been cured undoubtedly due to the Sister Kenny treatment, they wanted to meet me, to interview me and to invite me to a dinner for Sister Kenny. This got enormous publicity which I like to think was a help to Sister Kenny.

I never contributed to Warm Springs fund-raisers because they were denouncing Sister Kenny as a fake, and refusing to see that she was claiming to have a treatment for polio that relieved spasms, pain, and muscular atrophy. Sister Kenny was an Australian nursing sister who had to resort to her own ingenuity in nursing children who got polio in Australia's outback. She found that hot packs and physiotherapy when the disease first became apparent often resulted in healing the damaged nerves before they died. My left hand was useless, for instance, and I remember when a physiotherapist saw a flicker in my thumb, she urged me to concentrate on that spot, and to try to make it move. Countless repetitions, and it worked. Sister Kenny asked me about the onset of the disease. I told her about feeling as if I had stomach flu and that I stayed in bed for a day because I had a temperature. Since my temperature had gone the following day, I went canoeing. At supper that night I noticed I was developing a stiff neck. By the middle of that night the paralysis had started.

Sister Kenny told me that probably if I had just taken it easy after my "summer flu", I might never have experienced the paralysis.

There's no question I was burning my candle at both ends, so to speak, that summer of '42. I was acting in six out of eight plays at the Knowlton Playhouse. We were rehearsing one play and acting another at night. I also had a few boyfriends—typical behaviour of a seventeen-year-old. Lots of people in Knowlton had stomach flu two weeks before I got polio. It was thought that because I had recently come from England where polio was relatively unusual, that I had not built up an immunity to the poliovirus.

I had been taking art classes before I got polio. I think polio robbed me of some of my ambition. It must have taken a certain toll on my energy level too. I'd always been athletic and liked to excel in whatever I undertook, but after my recovery my ability to play a good game of tennis was shot and skiing became difficult because I could no longer put my full weight on my ski poles. Nor could I swim properly. And having thin shoulders, I didn't want to wear an evening dress that was too bare and show my protruding shoulder blade. I always wore a jacket.

I don't think my sister and three older brothers were affected by my having polio nor do I think polio has affected me too much either, although I do remember when my three children were young, having to take a day off just to sleep. My husband was supportive and always encouraged me into doing things. But when he died I then had to either sink or swim, and I discovered that I was able to swim. So for the last twenty-five years I've been very busy. I went to night school at McGill, got a certificate in management which I found quite easy, much to my surprise, and went to work for an appraiser who was hesitant about employing me because there weren't any women in the appraisal profession, except one friend. She was the head of relocation at Royal LePage and told me that if I got a job, she would give me work.

Not many people can tell I have had polio. It isn't really noticeable. Polio has left me with a weakness on my left side and back, and my voice is shaky, doubtless because I was in an iron lung. I nearly lost my voice then. I don't think I'm weaker over the years, even though I have lots of aches and pains of an arthritic nature. They have crept up gradually. Perhaps they result from polio. I am having a few problems with my neck. My posture is terrible, my back is sore, my feet bother me. I visited Dr. Trojan and her recommendation was for me to lose weight. I've lost fifteen to eighteen pounds in a year, but I haven't followed up on my breathing test yet. Perhaps I should.

I have always been right on top of any illness, or I think I have, and I've been very fortunate. My experience with polio has made me alert to my health needs.

I'm trying to slow down, not to do so much, and to find more time to paint.

Written in 1998, this text also incorporates Betty Goodfellow's contribution to "Nursing Highlights 1934 to 1960, Montreal Neurological Institute and Hospital".

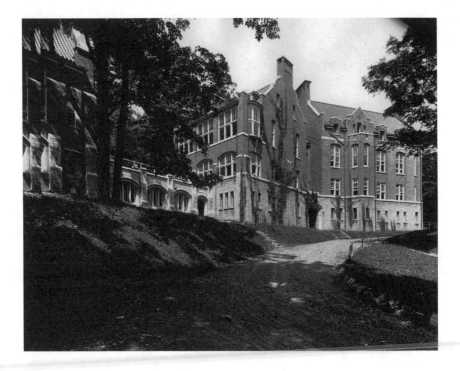

Children's Memorial Hospital, Cedar Avenue, Montreal, 1913.
Notman Photographic Archives.

I Didn't Let Polio Get in My Way

AUDREY McGUINESS

I WAS STRICKEN with bulbar-spinal polio in August 1942 when I was eight-and-a-half years old. Considering I was totally paralyzed, I had a remarkable recovery. I was in the hospital for eighteen months where, initially hot packs, and then physical and hydrotherapy were a daily routine. They wouldn't release me from the hospital until I could walk, but I still had to learn how to go up and down stairs. Eventually I learned to ride a bike, but not uphill. I tried downhill skiing once, but that just didn't work. I learned how to skate but could only go round corners one way; I just couldn't get my right foot over my left foot. My right side was, and still is, my weak side. I learned how to swim, but not for any distance or duration. I regained a lot of strength in my arms, legs, and back, but it certainly wasn't 100 percent. When I was older I took up cross-country skiing (I sat down on the hills), but there was no way I could ever play racquet sports.

But going back to the beginning of my life with polio—I'd been to a birthday party and coming home I suddenly felt so ill I thought I was going to die. That night the doctor came and did a lumbar puncture with me on the kitchen table. He took it off to have it analyzed. It was positive. He returned around midnight to take me to the Children's Memorial Hospital from Pointe Claire. I don't remember too much about the early days in the hospital. I was so out of it. But I do remember waking up and finding my legs propped up on pillows, and I remember being wrapped in hot packs, and I'll never forget the muscle spasms.

I was first admitted into Ward L. Then I was taken to Ward D and that is where I was when I got scarlet fever in March 1943, which meant I had to go to the Royal Alexandra Pavilion where I was in quarantine until I recovered from what turned out to be a mild case. The first night there I woke up screaming because I thought I saw a room full of ghosts. Apparently the ghosts were the nurses' quarantine gowns hanging up outside each cubicle and I wasn't pacified until they had all been removed! I think I took my first steps while there. My treatment wasn't interrupted during this period because a physiotherapist would come from the Children's to work with me every day. I also had an attack of appendicitis while in the hospital (I don't know when but before I could walk) and I was whisked off to the surgery ward where, for a week, every time the stretcher came into the room I thought it was for me. The only good thing about that week was that they fed me Jell-O and ice cream every day. When the stretcher finally did come for me, it wasn't to the surgery I went but back to my old ward. The neurosurgeons won out over the regular surgeons, persuading them not to operate and cut muscles that were beginning to recover. Why didn't someone tell me!! To this day I still have my appendix.

My doctors at the Children's were Drs. Struthers and Goldbloom. I remember Nurse Akagawa who was very nice. Everyone liked her. And then there was the head nurse, Miss Collins. Everyone was afraid of her, including the adults. There was a Miss Dickinson who went off to the war effort like so many nurses, and this was one of the reasons a lot of the nursing was done by volunteers.

Most of us who were hospitalized in the early 1940s with polio will remember the hot packs. The nurses would fill the old wringer washing machines with boiling hot water and put pieces of cut-up wool blankets into the boiling water. Using pincers they fed them into the wringer and then rushed them over to your bed and, piece by piece, covered your body. You were then wrapped in a blanket to keep the heat in. This was done two or three times daily.

We got up to all sorts of pranks in the hospital, like children everywhere. One morning I didn't want to wake up so I pretended to be sort of dead for what felt like eternity (maybe it was only for a few minutes!) surrounded by doctors prodding me. Eventually one doctor thought of tickling me and that spoiled my game. I remember when one of the older boys put me on a stretcher and whirled me around the room, knocking all the beds out of line, and another time when I had someone push two beds together so that I could play with my friend. I made the mistake of sitting in the middle where they joined and soon the beds split apart and I found myself on the floor unable to get up. That was the first time my kneecap went out of joint. It has since happened quite frequently. They just pushed it back into position! I also remember rocking myself around on a chair. We got all over the place that way. Those who could use their legs would push. I rocked. As for chewing gum, I haven't had a piece in my mouth since my hospital days. I was made to chew it constantly to exercise my jaw.

My parents would come to see me on Sundays without fail. And every Wednesday would find my mother visiting me. Those were the only visiting days. If she had a cold, she couldn't come inside, but would be at the window reassuring me she was there and that she really cared. I missed my brother and sisters. Children weren't allowed to visit in those days, only in the summer if we were in Ward L with its outside veranda and our beds were pushed outside so we could get some sun and fresh air.

My polio was undoubtedly a devastating blow to my parents. My mother not only had our family to care for, but also, for several extended periods of time, my aunt's two children (my aunt had multiple sclerosis). With so much activity going on, it must have been a nightmare for her. Although health insurance paid for some of my hospital and medical expenses, it must have been difficult on the family. We were four children, I being the second oldest. We think that my brother and sisters had polio too. They were sick with fevers but recovered.

When I left the hospital I had to go back for physiotherapy for a while, but I don't remember for how long, perhaps only for a month because it was such an arduous trip coming in from Pointe Claire. We didn't have a car during the war, of course, so we had to take the train, and a bus, and then finally a taxi to the hospital. My mother was eventually trained to give me exercises at home and so we no longer had that horrendous trip to the hospital. Although I do remember one exciting trip from the hospital to the CP train station in an ambulance—with the laundry! The driver drove all the way to the station with the siren on with me sitting up in the front seat!

I was allowed to go back to school at the beginning of April. Having been taught reading and writing and some math in the hospital, I was allowed to skip Grade 3 (my sister was in Grade 3 and I didn't want to be with her!) and go into Grade 4 for the last few months of the year. However, having virtually skipped two years of school, going into Grade 5 was very difficult for me (all that strange math—multiplying and dividing were Greek to me) and I had a lot of catching up to do in all my courses.

I don't think polio had too much of an impact on my childhood, at least not one that got in my way, except for sports. I was just too busy trying to catch up and getting on with my life. The other children in my neighbourhood accepted me as I was. The first realization I had that I wasn't exactly like all the rest was after the war when we were out on the baseball field with a new teacher. As I was running from home base to first base, he kept telling me to run faster. Of course, I couldn't run faster. I could barely run! Finally one of the kids told the teacher I had had polio and thereafter I was allowed to do my slow run to the base. That was the first time I can remember that someone had to be educated about my hidden disability. Another time, the girls were going off to another school to play basketball. I didn't want to stay in school with all the boys, so I walked to the bus, but instead of getting on, I just walked home. I was too shy then to ask what I was supposed to do.

What turned out to be post-polio syndrome started affecting me in 1976, thirty-four years after the original polio. But it wasn't diagnosed as such until many years later, after I had seen an article in the *Gazette* about post-polio syndrome, and after I had become involved with Polio Quebec Association and learned about Dr. Cashman and Dr. Trojan at the Montreal Neurological Institute and Hospital where they had developed a Polio Clinic.

I first experienced back problems when I was in my twenties, which were related to the scoliosis I had as a result of polio. Then in my early forties I was beset with severe back and neck problems. The pain went all the way up and down my spine, and into my neck. Because I was so afraid of what was happening, I wasn't walking very much. I couldn't. It was painful and it was winter and I was terrified of falling. I was eventually hospitalized in the neurological ward of the Montreal General where they did all sorts of tests to exclude the possibility of my having other known nerve-related diseases. I was sent home with the discouraging words, "You are doing really well considering your condition," but they couldn't tell me what my condition was. They might have had an inkling that it was related to my polio, but if they did, they certainly said nothing to me. They told me to start walking and suggested physio treatments. I started to walk again in order to strengthen my leg muscles which had weakened due to non-use that winter. But I kept having problems with my neck. The braces didn't seem to be helping at all. I was like a zombie from my stiff and spasmed neck. In the early 1980s someone suggested I try a chiropractor. I was reluctant but finally did and that's when I began to feel relief. Although physical therapy helped me regain some of my strength, it is the chiropractic treatments that really put me on my feet.

It's been over twenty years since all this started. In 1996 I acquired a wheel-chair, although the doctor had suggested I get one four years earlier. Similarly, with my back brace and two canes. I guess I'm a procrastinator when it comes to these things. Perhaps it's denying what my doctor thinks is best for me. It's not until the discomfort becomes unmanageable that I succumb to using the support devices and, sure enough, they help. One of the most disturbing aspects of post-polio is that I can no longer just walk out the door to do my shopping. I have to plan my outings along with my flow of strength, and I'm now dependent on my car for getting everywhere. But I'm adapting and remembering that because post-polio syndrome has slowed me down, it will take me twice as long to get places. However, so far I have managed to keep up with all my interests, such as bridge, quilting, painting, reading, traveling and, of course, my family and friends. I also was involved in putting Polio Quebec's newsletter together for about twelve years. I recently bought a new condo, but even more exciting is the fact that I retired in November 1998. I am blissfully happy about that and I am sure that at the end of each day I seem to have more energy than I did when I had to go to work every day.

Would my life have been different had I not had polio? It certainly didn't stop me from traveling and working my way around the world. And now with post-polio syndrome, well perhaps I unconsciously got involved with bridge, art, and quilting because they were things I could do without expending too much energy. I'm not really sure. I just let things happen.

I think having had polio undoubtedly made me more sensitive to other people's problems. Even though my handicap was virtually a hidden one for the first thirty years, and I didn't know other polios until more recently, I was nonetheless very much aware of the difficulties others had, especially, for instance, my friend Esmé in England who is a dwarf. Perhaps because of my handicap I see or anticipate when people need help more readily than others.

In summary, I have always enjoyed life and didn't let polio get in my way.

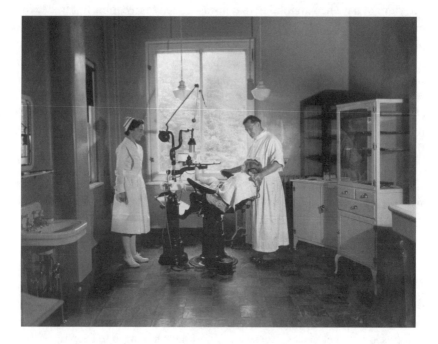

A visit to the dentist.
Shriners Hospital, Montreal.

From the Bombed-out Hospital in Stettin, Germany to Founder of Polio Quebec

Sieglinde Stieda

In the early 1980s Sieglinde Stieda spoke at a Montreal Rotary luncheon. She had taken time from her job as librarian at Société Radio-Canada to talk about polio and polios who thought their struggle with this disease was over. Sieglinde told the gathering about experiencing mysterious physical ailments including fatigue, pain, and weakness. This was before these symptoms were recognized as being possible derivatives of an old fight with polio, and a time when doctors were as perplexed, as were their patients, by questions about what was causing so much trouble for polios. Polios, like Sieglinde, felt that their problems were so severe that groups of them started gathering in cities across Canada to help each other cope with their new problems and to work together to get the attention of the medical community.

Rotarians in Montreal, Lloyd McLintock in particular, responded to Sieglinde by giving her about $200 seed money to pursue her search and to assist her in getting something started in Montreal that would address the new needs of old polios. By 1985 the group consisted of over 500 polio people. One of these members, a physician who lived outside Montreal, donated $500, which went a long way to pay duplicating and mailing expenses.

There was also the physiotherapist, the late Anne Marie Van Daele, who was most helpful in finding free meeting places and interpreting medical articles. Sieglinde also had help from the librarians at rehabilitation centres and medical libraries. She surveyed the medical libraries in Montreal and discovered that none had articles or books about polio beyond 1965. Her former boss, Bernard Bédard at the medical library at the Université de Montréal, became an invaluable resource. He also donated some pre-1965 polio books to Polio-Quebec. These Sieglinde gave to Monique Grégoire, a former scientist at the Université de Montréal.

Grégoire had broken her hip (polio weakness) and was using a wheelchair. At the time of the break she was treated with a medication that resulted in her becoming deaf. The medication was subsequently banned. But despite her various handicaps, including weak shoulder muscles, Mme Grégoire answered all the French telephone calls. She was able to hear with an amplified telephone. Since Sieglinde worked all day, Polio Quebec would not have got off the ground without the incredible dedication of Madame Grégoire and the late Joyce Jerret who answered the English queries. It was these two women who received all the telephone calls after every publicity campaign orchestrated by Sieglinde.[1]

When Sieglinde visited Dr. Baxter at the Montreal Neurological Institute and Hospital, she was quick to point out that research was needed as to why so many people were having new problems, stemming undoubtedly from their old polio. "If you learn more about this motor neuron disease," she said, "it might lead to discoveries that would benefit people with other puzzling motor neuron diseases." Dr Baxter confided that the Neuro had been thinking of putting together a motor neuron research group and that one of the young researchers they were considering hiring was Dr. Neil Cashman whose specialty was ALS and polio. Said Sieglinde, "The 500 members of this early Polio Quebec would be a possible research base for the Neuro. I don't think Neil Cashman ever knew the role I had played in getting him his job at the Neuro."

Sieglinde continues:

The first Polio Information document I wrote was under the guidance of Dr. John Dudley, a professor of neurolinguistics at the Université de Montréal. Among other things, John taught his students about the twelve pairs of cranial nerves. For several years I was John's teaching aide when he taught this subject to his huge classes (thirty to fifty students). I would lie on the desk and John would poke me somewhere and explain which cranial nerve was responsible for that particular movement. Thus, he showed them how my left 7th (facial) cranial nerve was paralyzed and how the 5th cranial nerve was weak. Students were also allowed to poke me.

In return for my help, John answered all my questions. He was a superb teacher and could make the most complicated article seem simple. He read whatever I gave him and explained what I didn't understand. I remember one evening in particular, John and his wife Rita had been in my apartment explaining an article on how the poliovirus kills off some motor neuron cells and how the orphaned muscle fibers send out distress signals and how, if enough healthy cells remain, the healthy cells send out "sprouts" to the orphaned muscle fibers. The light went on in my head and I remember pacing around my living room muttering, "I have to take care of my sprouts." Each year since I have learned more about what it really means "to take care of my sprouts" and my self-understanding has grown amazingly.

The other researcher who sent me in the "right" direction was Dr. William Rea of Texas. His seminal article was "The Environmental Aspects of the Post-Polio Syndrome".[2] Rea wrote, "Our work using the Environmental Control

Unit as a scientific basis for studies of chronic diseases suggested that perhaps some of the late polio problems might be due to an overload of environmental pollutants on wounded target organs."

He was supported in his theory by researcher Dr. André Barbeau. He told me about having done a study of the St. Lawrence Valley in relation to pollution there and the number of multiple sclerosis (MS) cases. He had found a correlation between the pollution levels and the number of MS cases. He told me that people were trying to suppress his study because the chemical companies in the St. Lawrence Valley did not want the information he had found to be known. Unfortunately Dr. Barbeau died a few months later. He had told me that he wasn't well enough to see me at the time.

However, his information and research certainly, in my mind, confirmed Rea's research. I have long been suspicious about the strange birth defects reported near a chemical plant in the St. Lawrence Valley.

Although I have never been able to travel to Rea's clinic in Texas, I am working with a physician who happens to have a degree in naturopathics as well. He persuaded me to avoid coffee and sugar, two major culprits. I also see another naturopath, Dr. Robert Ewing who introduced me to the idea of eating according to my blood type.[3] By following his advice I am able to control my springtime allergies. Dr. Ewing has a more sophisticated test that I haven't been able to afford yet. However, I have done chelation therapy using high doses of vitamin C. After the first three sessions of chelation, I was able to stop using enzyme supplements (I had terrible pains every time I ate). After the second set of three chelation sessions, I had an incredible surge of energy. However, along with the chelation, I need to take very expensive chlorella powder. The purpose of the chlorella and chelation is to pull mercury out of my body/brain. I can't really afford another three sessions, but I will take them again. It's sort of like insurance for me.

The increased energy does have drawbacks. I volunteer for too many committees and then the resulting paperwork overwhelms me and I have new "housekeeping", i.e., paper-pushing problems. However, I do enjoy my work teaching six-year-olds how to read. It's very satisfying. And if I can find a school district that will employ me after age sixty-five, I will continue working beyond that age. It gives me a lot of satisfaction.

Sieglinde recommends reading *Free To Fly–A Journey Towards Wellness* by Judit Rajhathy and books by Dr. Rea of Texas and books about healthy lifestyles (regular sleep, clean water, stress management such as acupuncture and massage, organic food, no evening meetings, etc.). By following these authors' advice and principles, as well as her own common sense, Sieglinde has been able to continue working full time. In reminiscing about her earlier experience with polio, she writes:

One of my most vivid memories of getting polio was seeing my siblings at the other side of a glass door and feeling frustrated that they were not allowed to come in. I had two major hospital stays as a toddler—polio in 1944 and typhus in 1945. An older brother was diagnosed with polio a week or two after me. We were in the hospital in Stettin, Germany at the same time. Stettin was a port city and was heavily bombed by the Allies during the Second World War. An older sibling has told me that every time there was an air raid the whole hospital was evacuated to a bomb shelter, except my brother Hansel and me. We were shoved into a dark cupboard. Parents were not allowed to visit, so when I was finally released, I did not remember my mother. However, apparently I remembered the shoes my mother held up.

Since it was wartime, I don't think I received any therapy or treatment. A year after getting polio I came down with typhoid fever. We were in a Danish prison/refugee camp where we stayed for two-and-a-half years. Only basic survival was possible at that time. From the fall of 1947 onwards when the family was returned to Germany, my mother dragged me to a lot of different doctors. Not until two or three years after immigrating to Canada did I get therapy. The physiotherapist came to our house and massaged my face with horrible smelling ointment. I hated the sessions. In 1958 Dr. Picard operated on me in Winnipeg, transplanting part of my thigh muscle to the left side of my face (known as a facial sling) and partially sewing up my eyelid.

I don't remember whether I was administered oxygen, but I did have bulbar polio and don't have full lung capacity now.

The impact of polio on my youth was unrelenting teasing and name-calling. I didn't even grow for two years. Although money wasn't an issue when I was young, it certainly is now. My commitment to the benefits of alternate health options comes at great expense; even dental expenses are high, for instance, due to difficulty of cleaning my teeth because of the muscle transplant. Conversion to amalgam-free fillings was also costly.

My five siblings had various feelings towards me. They thought I was spoiled and received preferential treatment. My mother couldn't even look at me without showing her pity for me. I hated this and left home because I didn't want to deal with her pity. My siblings found it difficult to believe these experiences were real, which added to my feeling of isolation from the family.

As an adult I have been called a high achiever. That was until I succumbed to post-polio syndrome symptoms and collapsed about twenty years ago. I was totally stressed out and unable to think and read. I had great difficulty walking. Finally, on March 1, 1981 I threw all my half dozen or so medications away, resulting in major withdrawal symptoms. I jogged for a while and started on the long road of learning what a healthy life style was like. I keep learning new things I can do for myself but I am finding most of these therapies such as chelation, massage, acupuncture, and organic food very, very expensive.

I have learned to moderate my lifestyle and expectations and now have lots of empathy for the less fortunate in life. In 1985, I started Polio Quebec.

Since it was my face that was visibly affected by polio, I noticed that even though most people treat me decently, there are some who have difficulty looking at or interacting with me. One boyfriend broke off with me, saying his mother or grandmother wanted him to date a normal looking young woman. Another boyfriend told me that he wanted to have a child with me but that he couldn't bear to wake up next to me and see my disfigured face.

At work, two young colleagues actually were so aggressive towards me that they hit me. The administration did nothing to discipline the two men. Neither did the union. Such physical or verbal aggression still happens occasionally, but not too often now.

Post-polio fatigue is the symptom that has most affected me—being unable to do all the things I want to do, or being unable to finish my PhD studies, as I just couldn't add all that academic stress to an already stressed body. Some people's reactions to me have also been disturbing, especially not being believed about my struggle with extreme fatigue. But I must admit that post-polio syndrome forced me to adopt a healthy lifestyle that has, it seems, worked well for me. Four of my five siblings had either cancer or cardio-vascular problems before the age of fifty. I am now sixty and comparatively healthy.

When my brother Hansel, who had polio at the same time as I did, died of a massive heart attack in the early 1980s, I remember thinking "I wonder if his death was related to polio?" Then I saw a polio article in the Montreal *Gazette* in the summer of 1984. I personally knew that stress had a connection to polio-affected areas of my body. In 1976 when writing a statistics exam I had terrible muscle spasms in my face. I don't know if these muscle spasms lasted two minutes, twenty minutes, or two hours, but I do remember holding my face and being embarrassed and frightened at the same time.

Starting a polio group in 1985 brought me into contact with other post-polio leaders. A few of us looked to non-allopathic medicine for answers and I am glad that we did, as this knowledge has greatly improved my quality of life. I'm still in contact with Bob Crout and his wife Grace in Ottawa. We continue to exchange thoughts on therapies, nutrition, research, and lifestyles. I am also indebted to Dr. William Rea of Texas whose research gave me the cognitive and philosophical basis of my new lifestyle.

The Honourable Paul Martins

Like Father, Like Son

PAUL MARTIN, JR. wanted to talk about his father, Paul Martin, Sr., because his father's life had been greatly affected by polio, whereas his hadn't. His father will always be remembered for the courageous stand he took to keep the Connaught Labs and their vaccination and dissemination programs going in the spring of 1955. The Salk vaccine had just been released, but in the United States, children were getting polio from it. The problem was traced to the Cutter lab in California. The urgency of combating this scourge had led to too much haste in production and it was discovered that the formaldehyde bath given the live virus for the vaccine was being withdrawn prematurely. The U.S. program was temporarily shut down. But Paul Martin, Sr., in his role as Minister of Health, was advised that the Connaught vaccine was safe, so he boldly gave the go-ahead for Connaught Labs to continue with its production and dissemination of the vaccine. Thus countless new polio cases in this country were avoided. It was a decision that took heroic courage on his part and confidence in his advisers. Had he misjudged, his career would have come to an abrupt end.

Paul Martin, Sr. played an important role in the Liberal ranks because of his impressive educational background in philosophy, international relations, and law. He had been appointed Parliamentary Assistant to the Minister of Labour in 1943. He entered the Cabinet in 1945 as Secretary of State and in 1946 became Minister of National Health and Welfare. In spite of the government's increasing conservatism on social issues, he managed to introduce a system of health grants, and by threatening resignation, made Prime Minister St. Laurent accept national heath insurance. This has been invaluable to all those with chronic illness, amongst whom are many old polio patients.

Long before Paul Martin, Sr.'s death in 1992, his genius for leadership was being equaled by his son, Paul Martin, Jr. Now Prime Minister of Canada, Paul Jr. said, "This is going to be a somewhat sketchy story because I had polio a long time ago, in 1946, when I was eight. I remember very little. There was a big epidemic in Windsor that year. In the summer of 1946 I was playing down at the beach. Coming home, I felt as if there was a plate in my stomach. My mother rushed me to the hospital."

In the 1940s polio put the fear of death into not only parents, but their children also. People would keep their distance in case the afflicted person was contagious, which left him or her with a terrible sense of isolation. However, Paul Martin Jr. remembers nothing like this. "Whatever they did to me in the hospital, I made a complete recovery, complete enough to be back in school after Christmas. I simply can't remember how long I was hospitalized, but am told that I had a very severe case of polio that affected my lungs. It was thought I wouldn't make it. I must admit that it is difficult to separate my personal experience back then from what my mother told me.

"I was apparently watched for two years; instructions had been given that I should never get upset. The end of this period signaled my last thought of polio until about seven years ago when Jan Brown, who was a Reform Member of Parliament and actively involved with post-polio, asked if I would like to go to a polio meeting in Ottawa to receive a commendation on behalf of my father from the Southern Alberta Post-Polio Support Society. Commendations were also being given that day to Dr. Salk and the Connaught Laboratories. This was the first time I had heard of the possible late effects of polio. It was at this Ottawa meeting in April 1995 that I recalled my memories of the disease for the first time in decades and saw personally by looking around the room that polio was still a challenge for many of the survivors, some of whom were affected by post-polio syndrome."

Asked if he remembered any particular anecdote related to his polio, following a pregnant pause, Mr. Martin recalled gleefully how his mother had been told that for the first two years of his polio he should never be upset. "But," said Paul Martin, "well do I remember when that two years was over. That was the end of my 'honeymoon'. She let it all out. I got absolutely killed for doing virtually nothing. Here's an example of how she spoiled me. I had lost a baseball. I remember losing it in a park, miles from home. It was my favourite baseball and I was devastated. Two days later, there was my baseball on the table. Years went by before my mother confided that she had bought a replacement for the lost ball and ripped off the cover to make it look authentic, all to appease me. I grew up like a pampered child for this period. I don't think my sister was jealous. She was so much younger."

When asked what impact polio had on his life, Paul Martin without hesitation was able to say, "I wish I could give you a deep insightful answer, but I don't really think it had any effect at all. I was fairly sick for about six months and was watched for a year and a half afterwards, and that was the end of polio for me.

"My Dad, on the other hand, was physically affected by polio. He was paralyzed down one side of his body, and was left with no sight in one eye and

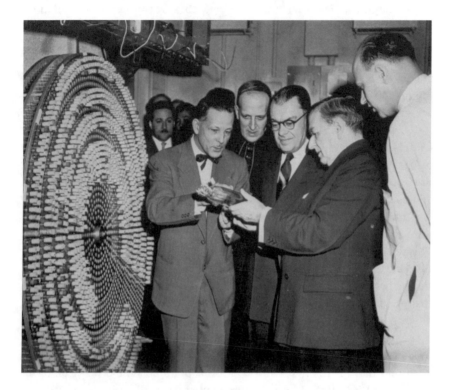

Inauguration of the polio lab at the Institut Armand Frappier, April 21, 1956,
for the production of the Salk vaccine.
Dr. Armand Frappier, Mgr. Irénée Lussier, Paul Martin Sr.,
Quebec Premier Maurice Duplessis and Dr. Vytautas Pavilanis beside
a rotating drum of vaccine.
Institut Armand Frappier.

a very weakened arm and leg. It wasn't really noticeable unless you were to see him in a bathing suit. As a child he managed to get everywhere, but only if pulled around in a cart or sleigh. He spent about two years coming back to a functioning level. He came from a very humble Irish/French family from the Ottawa Valley. It's quite conceivable that polio made him the man he was because he was the first ever in the family to go to university and he chose that route partly because more physical futures were incompatible, given his weakened body. My grandmother was without doubt a driving force in his life because she had been a teacher and was a very strong-minded person. In those days you could teach without special training. My dad attended Toronto University, Harvard, Cambridge, and Geneva Universities, and went on to lead a very public life."

Mr. Martin, Sr. spent thirty-nine years as MP for Windsor, Ontario, and as cabinet minister under Louis St. Laurent. Health was one of his many portfolios. He became connected to the March of Dimes in Ontario, for obvious reasons, and in 1994 the Paul Martin Senior Society was started. Monies collected went for medical research and the war against polio in particular. The Society honours those who share Paul Martin, Sr.'s vision and commitment. Since his brave decision in 1955 to carry on with the vaccine production benefited all of Canada, it might be a good idea to extend his Society and its goals across the country.

Some information has been extracted from the Ontario March of Dimes 2001 video *The Paul Martin Sr. Society: A Most Honourable Legacy*. The rest is from a conversation between the Honourable Paul Martin Jr. and Dr. Vitas Pavilanis who was director of vaccine production at the Institut Armand Frappier in Laval, Quebec.

I Feel Great When I Get up in the Morning

BERNADINE MARCHAND

I GOT POLIO IN 1948, at the age of thirteen, the year *South Pacific* came out. It's hard to understand why I was the one in the family to succumb to this disease when it was my older sister who was always getting sick.

We were in the Eastern Townships when polio struck, and were going black-berry picking. Feeling feverish, I didn't want to go, but my sister reminded me that we had to work for our room and board at my aunt's place while our parents were in Chicago. She said, "Come up the mountain with me and just sit quietly under a tree, and I'll promise to fill your pail." With this kind of help, my aunt didn't realize how ill I was.

Returning to Montreal from the country by car, I was unable to straighten up at the end of the trip, and passed out in the apartment. My mother hurried back from Chicago and rushed me to the hospital. I was totally paralyzed. Although I remember being given the spinal tap, I felt nothing. My pediatrician and good family friend Dr. Harry Bussière was my doctor. He persuaded my mother to keep me at home because the hospitals were overcrowded, while promising to visit me three times a day at home. He was true to his word.

Dr. Bussière's care was extraordinary. Singing tunes from *South Pacific*, he would focus his treatment on my legs, with hot and cold baths, and hot packs. I remember him trying every morning to push down my neck and that's when the pain would shoot down my spinal column. Needless to say, I didn't like this treatment, but he persisted until my neck got strong. After my baths, my mother and the doctor would wrap my paralyzed arms around their shoulders and walk me up and down the hallway with my legs dangling. It was extremely painful and I hated it. I remember the intense pain I had in my legs during the night. I slept in my mother's room (I don't know where my father slept during this period) and she would rub me with wintergreen. I can still remember the smell of that ointment.

My mother had never left us before that trip to Chicago, and she swore she would never again go away. Her love was very soothing and she was a fantastic nurse.

By February I was back in school, and I passed that school year. I graduated at age fifteen.

Post-polio syndrome crept up on me. I'd been married twenty-one years and had had six children. We lived in Hamilton, Ontario. Nobody there could understand the spasms that had started, the headaches, the weakness, and my not wanting to get up in the mornings. My body ached all over. I was sent to McMaster University Hospital where they put a cap on me with all sorts of needles stuck in my head. They did some tests with devastating results, i.e., showing that my muscles were deteriorating rapidly and that in two years, they reported, I would be totally paralyzed. That was in 1975.

My husband Roger's best friend's wife had contracted multiple sclerosis and he had left her. I don't know whether this is why Roger decided to leave me at a time when I needed him most, but he did. I loved him and thought our marriage was a good one. I worked for him at his very prosperous business. When he left me, it was cut and dried. No discussion. That was on December first—his birthday, and ninety-five people had been invited to his party.

He asked that I not live in Hamilton anymore, so I gathered the children and brought them crying all the way to my hometown in Montreal, and started a new life. I met a wonderful Ukrainian man. We married, had another child, but all the while the muscle spasms and headaches persisted. I'd learned to live with this and was relieved not to be paralyzed.

Once we had sold our two vegetarian restaurants in Montreal, we moved to Freligsburg. I worked at the Sutton Town Hall. It was a struggle making ends meet. Gene, my second husband, told me he had seen Dr. Gingras on TV. Dr. Gingras had been talking about post-polio syndrome, and it sounded similar to my problems. This was at the same time as the polio meetings were beginning in Montreal. I went to one at the late Joyce Jerrett's home. Although these meetings didn't change me, it was great to begin to understand what was happening to me, and to know that it wasn't all in my head.

Then I started to visit Dr. Cashman who prescribed the MRI (magnetic resonance imaging) tests. I never went on medication. After my husband died in 1994, I started using herbs more as a friendly gesture to a girl I liked than out of conviction they would do any good. These herbs were supposed to create inner balance. When I first took them, I broke out in a rash. My friend urged me to continue, saying that with these herbs old symptoms might come back and that I should not be afraid because they wouldn't come back again. There are two of these herbal products. One cleanses the bowel; the other rejuvenates.

I've been on the products now for four years. Within a month of taking them my headaches stopped, the arthritis in my hand stabilized, the muscle spasms left. Gone are the days when I would have to lie on the floor to get rid of these spasms. The only time they returned was in Mexico when in the ocean

I tried to fight a wave and moved in such a way as to provoke a spasm. I am now on a maintenance program. Dr. Cashman noticed the improvement in my condition.

I believe that when something is over, it's over. Perhaps I wouldn't be able to say this if it weren't for what I learned with my PPS experience. I had a very bad kidney at one time. I was on cortisone. They were waiting to put me on the dialysis machine and I had even put out a call for donors. But I recovered. They wondered what I had done. Simply put, I woke up in the middle of the night and ate a whole bottle of Bovril. I hadn't had salt in over a year. Suddenly my condition changed. I don't know why. There were certainly many people praying for me. Prayers, love, looking for new avenues of openness, coupled with hard work and good medical practice (perhaps even Bovril!) all play their part in recovery. But now that is behind me. I think I have also conquered the threat of post-polio syndrome, if not entirely, by about 80 percent. I no longer have spasms. I feel great when I get up in the mornings and I don't have headaches.

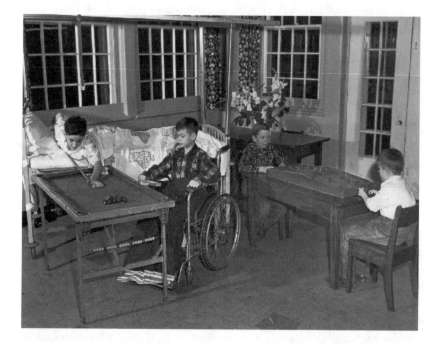

The games room.
Shriners Hospital, Montreal.

Thrown a Curve

LOUISE STOCK

I WAS BORN IN MARCH 1949, the first of eleven children. When I was two months old polio struck. I had countless orthopedic interventions, but it wasn't until I was eight that I underwent a major surgical correction for my polio scoliosis deformity. I should stand 5'6", but measure barely five feet. My right hip is higher than the left, I have a hump on my back by my left side, and my thoracic area is stunted due to the scoliosis, therefore I have learned to dress so that my clothes camouflage the curvature of my spine. Nonetheless, throughout my life I have been treated normally by almost everyone. No preferential treatment, and I am grateful for that.

Now that I am in my fifties, I am aware that much of my fatigue and decreased endurance undoubtedly come from my polio, and this has forced me to adjust my life so that I get enough rest. I have also been left with reduced sensation below the neck on the left side of my body, and this is quite unusual.

According to old hospital records and my parents, I was seen at the Montreal Children's Memorial Hospital on May 3, 1949, with a fever and abnormal behaviour for a baby of two months. While being bathed, it was noted that my right leg when raised fell lifelessly. It was thought to be a virus, but polio wasn't suspected until the fall. So I was sent home. Within a week I was back in the hospital. Still no diagnosis or treatment. Home again. By September there was evidence of dorsal scoliosis and it was only then the doctors assumed I had polio. When I started walking at ten months my parents noticed that my curvature was getting worse.

Records in the following decade show over thirty hospital visits and approximately twenty-one admissions lasting from two to twenty-four days, first at the Children's Memorial on Cedar and then at the Montreal Children's on Tupper. Basically I had X-rays, neurological tests, general evaluations, and the application or the removal of plaster thoracic casts or laced removable lighter-weight jackets, which fitted around the entire thoracic area from below the armpits to the groin area. Many of the procedures that required hospitalization then would be done as an outpatient today. Doctors seemed to be learning as they went.

Up to age six I was fitted with a sequence of plaster casts, attempting to correct my curvature. Some were applied too snuggly to allow for stomach expansion after eating, therefore often requiring reapplication. I was made to stand on a wooden stool a few feet off the ground with a suspended noose, which acted as a harness. It would be put around my chin and head and cranked upwards to straighten me vertically. This meant I would be standing on my tiptoes on a stool. The cast was then applied. The soft ribbed inner cotton stretchy cloth was covered by warm wet plaster rolls smoothed out to harden. Often the casts wore sores under my armpits, or in the hip or groin area. They would cut the plaster at the top of the cast, and then fold over the last bit of the white cotton lining and get some white plaster to make a nice smooth edge. But when cutting the top of the plaster cast, plaster crumbs would fall back under the plaster cast which would irritate me. When I got home, we'd take a vacuum cleaner with a nozzle and clean me up, just like I was returning from the beach full of sand. My favourite cast was the lightly laced Riser cast that I could remove to go swimming. Swimming is now my main form of physiotherapy.

My hospital experiences were generally good. My word was valued in treatment, so I was often asked to try, or I volunteered, or my parents volunteered me with my approval, for experimental procedures and techniques. I thank my parents for giving me a positive outlook on everything. I was brought up to help, and to be caring and sociable at home, and these were useful traits for life in the hospital. I took part in the passing out of food trays, picking up toothbrushes and handing out baking soda paste, even helping the nurses make beds with hospital corners. I was in fact repeating the work there that I had been doing at home. It was a close-knit group in that old hospital, like a family. Everybody seemed kind. The tooth fairy often remembered to put money under my pillow when one of my teeth came out.

Happiness in the old Children's hospital was being able to go out on the big verandah where there were always lots of people. I remember thinking mealtime was like a party. There were even snack times with juice and graham wafers. Although there was a set schedule, just like home, life in the hospital was never dull. They would even tune into CJAD Radio so we could hear the music that sent children marching off to school. We were witness to lots of funny things in the hospital—kids ripping their clothes off, mixing bowls of food together, people visiting and bringing gifts, the kindness of the staff. I remember everyone smiling, although down deep are hidden the more traumatic memories of suffering and even deaths.

If you needed any special treatment, you were taken by stretcher to another building. The stretcher was held by two porters who would make me feel as if I were going for an exciting ride as they bumped me down the many stairs.

Even though I was strapped on, I would often slip. In a small way, they would turn an ordinary trip into an adventure.

I was a patient again when the hospital moved into its new quarters on Tupper. That was exciting. Everything was fresh and clean. We were even shown movies. Woody Woodpecker ones were the most frequently shown. I remember the movie man. He had great rapport with the children. There were lots of toys and tricycles, even visiting rooms. The toilets and sinks were at children's level. It just seemed like a big playhouse. Even the staff's spirit was better. It was a new environment and inspired great plans for the future.

I really sympathized with the nurses who had to deal with so many young children. Particularly difficult was getting patients to take their medication. I couldn't swallow pills and to this day I have a high gag reflex. The nurses thought that the best thing for me would be something sweet, so they mashed the antibiotic into some jam to mask it, but that was worse. I remember being coached to swallow because if I brought up the pills, I would have to take them again. There was a lot of projectile vomiting on the ward, provoking screams and crying.

Dr. McIntyre and Dr. Sugar did my spinal surgery. The latter we called Prince Rainier because he looked so much like the Prince of Monaco. In February 1957 I had a Hibbs and Abbe fusion using bone from the Montreal General Hospital bone bank. The only complication was a headache!

Once, when I tried to get the nurses to do something about the boy who was crying in the bed across the room, they gave me a needle instead of him!

I've been stoic in the face of pain, having been coached early on by my parents to be brave. Also, Sisters of the Holy Cross used to visit me and we would pray together. Some pretty miserable things were done to me, but a minimum of drugs kept me feeling terrific after surgery. Or was it the power of prayer? A miracle? Who knows!

One of the times I had excruciating pain was during a myelogram the day before surgery when I was eight years old. I was on my stomach. The needle broke in my back when the doctors were marking the place on my spine where the surgery would be done. A piece remained. They were unsuccessful in extracting it and it was agony until the next day when I had a spinal fusion from D4 to L2. The surgeon gradually straightened my spine by fusing eleven vertebrae, hoping this would resolve my double scoliosis. I returned from post-op heavily drugged with a type of turtle shell on my back. I said, "Hi," to my parents and proceeded to ask for my schoolbooks. I was then put in a room and tied down with a restraining jacket covering the hips, the chest, and the shoulder/neck area. I requested this latter one be undone and promised never to move. I was soon placed on a Stryker bed, similar to the one John F. Kennedy had used after his back accident. It was on a frame, supported at each end by a swivel mechanism. To turn me over they would put the bottom layer on top, like a sandwich, rotate me, and then remove the top layer, which would put me on my stomach looking through a padded hole. The first time they tried it, I fell out sideways onto the floor so then a sheet was used like a safety ribbon. This frequently had me looking downwards during visiting hours. I remember this distinctly, because my parents asked that the rotation be arranged so that I could look up during visiting hours at least once during the day.

I was a very active child, and here I was, bedridden. My major entertainment when looking up was counting the holes in the acoustic ceiling. When people came they would ask me what number I had reached! I was rewarded with cashews—my favourite nuts—milkshakes, and lots of cards, flowers, and drawings from my classmates. Dad also came by religiously after work downtown, always leaving off more film for the camera he had left me. Being an A student and wanting always to forge ahead, I worried about missing school. My parents arranged for the hospital to school me and forwarded assignments.

I left the hospital by ambulance with a heavy thoracic plaster cast and had to remain prone for nine months. My parents set up a bedroom in the living room. A mirror was set up on the wall so that I could always feel included in what was going on. I could even see into the kitchen. Getting a little restless in the summer, I remember trying to get up and stand when nobody was looking. But I didn't realize how heavy the plaster cast was. I got caught. That wonderful mirror did me in!

Meanwhile medical expenses were covered by my Dad's Blue Cross policy. The only problem was that he was constantly filling in forms. He tried to find funding for a number of projects, one of which was an intercom system that would connect me at home to my classroom while I was bedridden. Even though the equipment was available, we never got the project off the ground because of local community politics.

My parents always did their best to help me feel part of family life. I especially remember the kitchen table Dad had made that was level with the sink. I could lie on it to do the dishes and feel I was doing my share of household chores. They also adapted an appliance dolly to take me to the beach. In my bathing suit, with or without my cast on, some children would make comments about my crookedness. I only remember thinking that it was strange they didn't have casts too. I certainly don't remember ever being ostracized.

By September my cast was replaced by a lighter one, but I was in trouble. Soon after coming home, I began to feel quite ill. I was feverish and a strange odour was coming from my cast. This cast had been experimental. To be fitted, I was laid flat on a very narrow board. There was a noose or harness around my neck, and my legs were taped. Then a person at either end cranked me to straighten out my body as if I were a piece of taffy. Plaster was applied, first the soft lining, then the wet plaster. How I loved the smell of it! I complained right away that the cast felt too tight, and even whimpered, but the conclusion was that it was okay. I kept complaining that the cast was pressing on the hump so tightly it had worn my skin raw and I was stuck to the inner lining. The cast had to be sawed off, except for a small circular piece on the hump area which had to be soaked off gradually with compresses. I finally healed, got a replacement cast, but was left with a wide oval scar on my hump. Eventually I had to learn how to walk again. It made me feel a little low because my legs just wouldn't move the way I wanted them to. Finally it all came together.

I was surprised one snowy November evening to be told by the doctors I could go home. That was it. I wouldn't have to come to the hospital any more. I phoned home but my Dad said it was too late to come and get me, knowing very well that Mom was on her way, having been already notified that I was to be discharged. Within a few minutes of the phone call, Mom surprised me. There she was at the hospital doorway. I saw her at this joyous moment as a real angel from God. It was one of my closest moments with her; it still brings tears to my eyes. She took me in a taxi to Central Station and we went home by train to St. Laurent. The very first thing I did was to have the best bath of my life. Dead brown flaky skin came off, but the cast was gone now and forever. I loved my Mom so much for coming that evening, while Dad stayed home with the six other children. My parents always found time to be nice to me.

Did my polio affect the family? My parents bravely say no. They were good Catholics and took things as they came. I had six other brothers and sisters when I was seven. The last two were identical twin girls. All through that time my parents still planned to have twelve children. They felt that if they could afford them, why not have them? They waited five years and had three more boys and another girl. Not one of all these children reacted to me as an ill person, doubtless because my parents treated me normally. I believe I am the wiser and happier for it.

When I had my last hospital check-up in 1959, polio had little effect on my life. I had no trouble as a youth with summer employment. I was never refused an application due to physical handicaps. As a teen, I felt discomfort only once, and that was in a line-up at Expo 67 when a young person said something about a freak. I sloughed that off as an insensitive remark.

When baby-sitting some children one winter, a little one patted my hump and exclaimed, "Louise, your shirt's bunched up under your sweater." I acknowledged this bit of information, and that was the end of that. I was apprehensive about going to college, knowing it would be competitive and that there would be dating. But I had somehow learned to be at ease with people, and they with me. There was always a group around me. I went to fraternity parties and dances. In fact it was at college that I met my husband. I was quite flattered when friends would ask me what I did to attract so many young men when they couldn't get a date. I explained to them that you just have to be yourself.

I married my college sweetheart Richard and had two beautiful daughters Erin and Melissa. But prior to each delivery, they would hospitalize me two weeks in advance, hoping to provide the right conditions for a safe vaginal delivery and avoid a Caesarean section. I was subjected to lots of tests, pelvic measurements, and monitoring. I had three false labours for each delivery. The doctors counseled against my nursing the babies. They felt I wouldn't be strong enough.

My work experience began in Student Services at Vanier College and then I moved on to the Counseling Department as a paraprofessional. At college I steered towards social work, but was told I would burn out quickly because I took too much to heart. Sure enough after a few years in the counseling department I was ready to move on to academic and vocational counseling. One year later I transferred to John Abbott College. After my first child I had hoped to return to work, but my stamina wasn't up to being both a mother and working outside the home.

In my community with other young moms there were many times when I felt I wasn't fully accepted. A friend would tell me that someone was uncomfortable being with a handicapped person. This was usually at a sandbox or in the park. The interesting aspect of the fickleness of some people is when they found out which house I lived in or which car I drove, or how well off I was, everything would then be okay. This was hard for me to fathom, having gone through all that I had. I realized that they could only draw on their life experience. Most people did not realize I was handicapped when they first met me, and then would be taken aback, putting their arm around me for instance. Then they would comment on how well I camouflaged my hump. A couple of times people withdrew from me feeling creepy about my unusual posture. I would also be aware of my scoliosis in doctors' offices where there were other people with handicaps, but they seemed much worse off than I was. I knew I was fine because I skated, skied, swam. I did everything I wanted except horseback riding. My children got used to my need for rest and my being unable to be as active as other moms. They were brought up to help out a lot. They seem well adjusted, even proud of me, and often wrote of their admiration in school essays.

Now that my life is a bit quieter and my children are grown up I'm aware of being generally fatigued particularly after a major project. I used to attribute this feeling to keeping a large house and raising a family and to my A-type personality. The body seems to say, "Enough" at a certain point. It's like being on a boot camp survivalist expedition, and completely collapsing from exhaustion. The odd time there seems to be a bit of nausea and the need to sleep a little in the afternoon, about twenty minutes. If I miss that I go around feeling sort of thickheaded, unable to concentrate. After all, quality time is more important than quantity. I keep a long and active day, always curious and on the move. But I've recently given up cross-country skiing and going out in the evenings. I'm just not the person I used to be.

My curvature complicated a gall bladder operation. The surgeons discovered the organs weren't where they expected them to be. They had to clamp me into a position, which left me with a lot of post-operative discomfort. After surgery I started choking and was having trouble breathing. A few years later, following a procedure to retrieve a gallstone, the drugs administered had me walking in a dream-like state around the hospital floor one night. No one noticed that I had gone to the nursing station and taken slips of paper. In the morning I found some nurses' recordings of patients' vital statistics and stuffed them into my dressing gown pockets. I think these unusual reactions undoubtedly had something to do with my reduced lung function and the effect of the anesthetics. Drugs have always been a problem. Even a Gravol pill will knock me out for three hours.

My curve felt much worse after the gall bladder operation. Both inside and outside, I felt unbalanced. I would put my right hand on my hip to keep myself straight, or sometimes even over my head just to balance myself and relieve that feeling of going crooked. I'm told that it was merely a question of muscles realigning themselves and that I would get used to it. Sure enough, I did.

A tedious problem these days is to find suitable clothing as I age with my deformity. The right side of my body, specifically my shoulder area, is a little atrophied, which means clothing is a problem with the right arm hole, and the curve on the right side makes the hip more prominent. This means I have to try on many items before I find something that fits. It's an activity that I do only on my own. When I have to put aside one piece of clothing after another because they don't fit, the salespeople wonder what is wrong with me. The word "polio" has little meaning for them these days, although they are very understanding once told, and allow me into changing rooms with armfuls of garments.

It was also important to me that my children not become insecure about their mother's handicap. I didn't want them to think I might be unable to look after them or that their maternal safety net would let them down. I learned that my mother had reassured them years ago that if anything were to happen to me, she would look after them.

Polio has been a major player in making me the person I am today. It has made me more compassionate and appreciative. It is a real learning game. I'm fully aware that if you have your health, you have everything. It has also given me the opportunity to meet lots of people, including the Queen and Prince Philip in 1959 when they visited Montreal to open the Seaway. I was chosen to present the Queen with a bouquet on behalf of the Montreal Children's Hospital. Thinking it unfair that Prince Philip wasn't going to get anything, I took a new wallet my father had brought home and hid it away so that I would have something suitable for the Prince. But my plan was discovered with a gentle reprimand from my parents who could hardly be too angry once they knew why I was in effect stealing the wallet. A *Gazette* reporter heard about this story and suggested I cut a rose from the bouquet I was to give to the Queen, place it back in the bouquet and when the time came to present the bouquet, I could then reach into it and give the Prince the severed rose. This I did, saying to him, "This is for you, Prince Phillip, you never get anything." Cameras flashed and people clapped, and my picture appeared worldwide. It was a very special day for me.

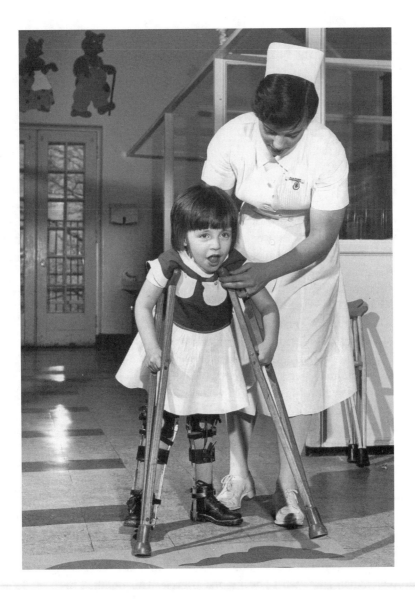

The challenge of walking with two sets of braces.
Shriners Hospital, Montreal.

There Are Many Negative Things in My Life that I Turned into Positives, Like My Handicap

Maurice Lwambwa-Tshany

I was born in Lumbumbashi, Congo (Zaire). I was struck by polio when I was two years old. The disease caused panic and distress at home. There was no word like "polio" in Africa; one simply said, "It was due to the needle given by the nurses." After the acute phase of the disease I moved around on all fours. My two lower limbs were affected. My parents did what it took to get me to a point where I could walk with crutches. They took me to an orthopedic centre daily.

The therapists gave me some kind of apparatus to try to help me get around, but I had already developed such skill moving around on all fours that I quickly put them aside. I was very obstinate, and besides, I found the apparatus did more harm than good. I was just fine with four legs.

I moved very quickly and I played outside like everyone else. It should be said that the attitude in Africa is not like that in Canada. The other children found it normal to see me moving on all fours because they all knew that I could not walk. My parents treated me like my brothers and sisters, but obviously I could not wander too far from the house. There was a certain parameter within which I was allowed to play with the neighbours, and if I ventured beyond that limit, there was hell to pay.

I had a chance to go to school because it was very close, just a few minutes from the house. I never needed to cross the street. For my first and my second year I went to school where my father was teaching. At this time I did not even own a wheelchair. Sitting on a bicycle, I was brought to school by my older brother. When I was ten I got my first tricycle. This one had been made in Belgium especially for handicapped children and allowed me to pedal with my hands. It was then that I became completely autonomous since I could go anywhere and when I wanted. Obviously, many places were not accessible to handicapped people, but at this time it wasn't better or worse than any other country. I always climbed steps on four legs.

There was a time when I was placed with a religious community to give my mother a rest. I stayed there for one year. My parents often came to visit me. I was with other children like myself, and don't have any bad memories from this stay with my new extended family. After I returned home I progressed like other children. We were ten boys in our family and I was the third child. My mother taught us to do the housework and each of us, including me, did his share. We had only two sisters. They were students at a boarding school and they didn't grow up with the family.

The fact that I had polio did not harm my life as a child. I led a completely normal family life. I shared activities with my brothers and I even played soccer on all fours. It was as if I had forgotten my legs. For me, in my head, I walked. I played soccer with normal people, but I hit the ball with my hands and that was acceptable.

There was a time when charlatans were rather popular in Africa. They claimed to be able to cure any disease, it didn't matter which one. My mother wanted to consult these people. One quack had her believing that I would be able to walk in fifteen days. Eventually my father decided enough was enough and that my mother should not trust these people anymore. Apart from the charlatans, I did not undergo any other treatments.

In Zaire, now called the Congo, there was state medical insurance, but for my father who was a teacher and therefore middle class, there were no privileges in spite of his large family. I think that, all the same, he was able to face the extra expenses without too much difficulty.

I attended school like any other young person. In secondary school it was necessary to learn a trade. My father wanted me to be a shoemaker or an office secretary. I decided to investigate the Fine Arts School and when I touched modeling clay, I immediately fell in love with the material. I became a sculptor. It's not easy work. But even if I sell nothing during an exhibition, the contact with the public offers me all kinds of other opportunities.

Everyone knows that couples have their arguments or storms. There were conflicts between my parents. I remember one sentence that my mother often repeated: "I could never leave and abandon a sick child." My father understood. My mother had sworn never to abandon me, moreover, never to leave the family hearth. I was too young to grasp the importance of that sentence, but at the same time, it left an indelible mark on my soul. My mother is still alive today, but my father died a few years ago from cancer.

I never concerned myself about the future after becoming an adult. My parents always knew that without a career I would be unhappy in life. I have earned my own living through my art and I live like everyone else. I never had difficulty being with people. I greatly respect others and have found my place in society. If someone does not like me, I do not believe that it is because of my polio, but it is more that one single person cannot like everyone. If someone gives an opinion about me such that he doubts my abilities, I confront that opinion with, "You have illusions. I am married. I have children. I work."

"You have children? Handicapped children?" they ask me sometimes.

We have to face these prejudices. I have learned how to understand these reactions that in fact are based only on ignorance. In life everything depends on respect one for another.

Meeting girls during adolescence obviously demanded a lot of effort, but I have managed to do quite well because I have a lot of confidence in myself. I always had the company of girls. If I was hung out to dry with a refusal, I would go and sit beside a beautiful girl, the girlfriend of my friend for example, and I would act as if she were mine. Then the one that refused my advances would tell herself, "What? I told him no and she, who is more beautiful than me, tells him, 'Yes.' Am I an idiot?" I have always used this tactic and I have succeeded in having the company of beautiful young women.

I lived in a rural area. I used to travel to the airport with friends and when the planes arrived we would invite the stewardesses to go out and voilà!

I had a job and with the fruit of my labours I bought cool shirts like my buddies and entered into the competition. Life is a competition, is it not?

I arrived in North America in 1990, without my family. I met many people and in 1993 my beautiful wife Isabelle and my three children joined me. Two sons have since been born in Canada. I had a few problems at the beginning. The French I spoke was the French of France, and it was different from French that we speak in Quebec. For my children, it was inevitable they would speak Québécois. Sometimes I correct my daughter but she answers me, "Dad, don't forget, I am Québécoise." My daughters are able to tell the difference between the two languages, the French which we speak at the house and the French that they speak on the street.

Ever since living here, I have often been invited to schools to participate in conferences and inevitably I must answer many questions about my handicap such as when did I first get polio, if I am married, and if I have any children. To give the young people the idea of the value of the respect for life, I say to them, "Imagine me, a Black in a wheelchair, an artist-sculptor, and I have visited the White House with the organization Very Special Arts." With that the sun shines for everyone.

One day a young girl asked me, "Maurice, if someone gave you the choice of the use of your legs or to remain the way you are, which would you pick?"

I told her I would not choose to recover my legs at my age. I have overcome my limitations and have accomplished many things. It is the battle that I have won. I am okay like this. "And, if I had strong legs, I would not be here in your class today, would I?" I have overcome my handicap. I was handicapped as a young person, which has its own problems, but I turned things like my handicap into positives.

I always respect others, and often they respect me. There are times when someone may stand back looking embarrassed or uncomfortable in front of me. It seems, I have learned, I always have to take the first step. Sometimes I feel compassion for certain people when this is not out of pity, otherwise I move on.

Whatever the country of adoption, the lifestyle is always different. It is necessary to learn how to recognize the differences. When I arrived here I was ready for the challenge. I was not disappointed or put off by the differences because I had prepared myself for them. Certainly if I do not want to upset others I have to discard some of my former habits. When I go to visit my friends and there is a staircase, I do not embarrass anyone by going up and down on all fours. That could shock some people, even disturb them, or cause them to take pity on me. Those who feel uncomfortable and embarrassed form one of the barriers that society imposes on me. As I do not want these people to feel guilty, I avoid visiting them. As mentioned previously, I got around almost all the time on all fours when I lived in Africa. When I arrived here, it was a big lifestyle change for me to be constantly confined to my wheelchair.

I am still working a lot. Recently I have felt tired. I do not take painkillers, but when I am in pain or feel tired, I take vitamins. There are people who do nothing and are tired anyway. Sometimes I have to nap during the day; it is not because I am getting old! Everybody needs rest. I am a self-disciplined soul and I have to deal with post-polio syndrome, and that means rest and a little exercise to get the blood flowing and to preserve flexibility.

Without my handicap, perhaps I would have been an athlete. Also, I would have enlisted in the army for mandatory service. There is one thing for sure, however, I would not have made a career in art as I have done. As such, my handicap influenced my choice of career.

Today I like to get involved with community organizations that meet my needs at home. I believe in teamwork. I like to talk and exchange ideas, and I hate being isolated. It is true that I only work in my workshop, but this is ultimately to share with others.

Maurice Lwambwa-Tshany had a studio in Montreal. He exhibited in France, Italy, Brazil, U.S.A., Austria, Hungary, and Canada. He died in 2002.

Society Doesn't See Us as Normal Human Beings with Feelings, Hopes and Dreams

Daphne Dale-Bentley

At the age of twelve, on September 15, 1951, I was stricken with polio. It affected my whole body and has left me with next to no function from the waist down. My arms are basically strong, although fragments of muscles are missing here and there. I get around in a wheelchair—an electric one outside the home. And since my mother died, I live alone.

My full-blown polio was preceded by my feeling sick and hurting all over. The worst were my headaches. But I went to school anyway. I came home, and because I ate a huge lunch, Mum doubted me when I said I didn't want to go back to school. How could I be sick if I had eaten so much! So off I went, feeling wiped out. I was too afraid to tell my male teacher, fearing he would think I had my period. By the time I got home it was obvious from my appearance that there was something dreadfully wrong.

The doctor came and said "just growing pains ... go to bed and rest." Dad went away for the weekend to our remote country place in the Laurentians, having been reassured by our doctor that there was nothing to worry about. But at about 11 o'clock that Friday night, the paralysis started settling in. I kept trying to do things realizing all the while that I couldn't. I managed getting up to go to the bathroom, until the third time I fell and had to crawl back to bed. The final time, about three in the morning, I wasn't able to even raise myself off the toilet. I fell onto the floor and crawled to my mother. She called the neighbours who advised waiting until the morning. They came over at about seven to accompany us to the hospital. By then I was totally paralyzed. They carried me out to their car and took me to the Children's Memorial Hospital where I had a lumbar puncture. The diagnosis was polio. I was whisked away and quarantined at the Alexandra Pavilion until October 2, when I was returned to the Children's. What a wonderful place. It became my second home for three years. I was in Ward K—one of the hospital's huts on the side of Mount Royal. Fascinated by nursing procedures, and the doctors, I was always eager to help the head nurse. If she needed to know whether so-and-so had had physio, or an X-ray, or whatever, I always seemed to know everything that was going on! I must admit to being spoiled by nurses and doctors alike.

I don't have good memories of hot packs, though. Often they were left on too long, until they got cold and soggy, though I presume they helped. And I was really sensitive to touch. My first physiotherapy was in the hospital in the central building, but a year later I went to the recently opened Constance Lethbridge Centre, by ambulance, three times a week. After about a year and a half of therapy, they tried getting me to walk with leg braces, but it took two people to get me up between the walking bars. I knew it wasn't going to work, but didn't want to disappoint the physios. Finally, everyone agreed that a wheelchair was the answer. I've always worn a back brace. It helps support me. I can't breathe properly when I'm sitting up if I'm not wearing it.

Constance Lethbridge was there at the time, a wonderful woman who took a personal interest in each one of us. She was a large woman, and I'll always remember her beautiful flower-bedecked hats. The Centre started out in the Seminary School at McGill on University Street. From there they moved behind one of the breweries. Now of course they are on the western end of de Maisonneuve. The occupational therapist Dorothy Barrett was very special and we remained friends until her tragic death. It's awful, but I don't remember the names of any of my physiotherapists, probably because of my original experience with physio at the Children's Memorial Hospital. One of the physios there used too much force in an attempt to straighten my stiff knees. It was agony and caused me to have huge swollen knees for over a month. So even though I hated having physiotherapy, I knew it was important. I tried my best.

Mum used to visit me every single day. She told me later that she saw and treated this as a job. My father would come on weekends or drop by on his way to the Armory. After a year I asked my Mother not to come so often because I had developed a busy hospital life. She must have been quite relieved. So she came three times a week and on weekends. For three years I was virtually cut off from my friends. My dog was allowed to visit, though, as long as she stayed outside on the balcony.

There were quite a few Inuit children who came from up North. One little girl, Susie, just couldn't stop crying. But I adored her, and the feelings were mutual. She would eat for me, but for nobody else. There were a couple of Eskimo boys who used to love pushing me around in my chair. One day they were feeling mischievous and they pushed me right off the verandah.

I remember Christmas in the hospital. We all went over to the main building at the Children's Memorial. Our parents were allowed to be with us. The hospital really outdid itself. But the most exciting memory is that of the guppies given to me by a friend of my father's. Everyone looked after them.

The female guppy became pregnant, and when she gave birth I let out a yell. Everyone came running to witness all these little things being born. The next Christmas I was all set to go home when there was an epidemic of infectious hepatitis on the ward. I spent Christmas at the Alexandra in quarantine.

Discovering my sexuality while hospitalized had its problems. It was embarrassing to have the facts of life explained to me by a young intern when I got my first period, and humiliating to have another intern draw nipples and underarm hair on my cast and body with a blue pen. It made everyone laugh. But I was humiliated.

I used to write skits for the nurses and doctors which they would act out at Christmas time. I remember the mounted policemen who patrolled Mount Royal. They would take kids for horseback rides. I couldn't go because my balance wasn't good enough. It was only after about eighteen months that I could sit up, and then for only ten minutes at a time. My scoliosis was relieved by a special brace that held me up.

I was taught in the hospital by an absolutely wonderful teacher—Margaret Ellis. I loved her. As soon as I was able to hold a book, I became a voracious reader. Being in the hospital with mostly younger kids, I missed growing up with my peers, but I learned other things from hospital life. When it came to going home at age fifteen, I was terrified. I had lived in a protected world where I was totally accepted. But after two weeks at home, you couldn't have dragged me back! My old friends all came to visit me and took me places. Dad was great about adapting the house for me.

Polio had a major impact on my parents too. Shortly before I contracted polio, my parents had sold our house in preparation for a move to California where my father already had a job. Needless to say, we didn't go.

I went briefly to the School for Crippled Children before having to return to the hospital for another two and a half years for a spinal fusion. Because I was so tall, it had to be done in two phases. Dr. Murray McIntyre was my wonderful orthopedic surgeon. My family members in California knew Dr. Stryker (known for the Stryker bed), so when he visited Montreal my parents and doctors sought confirmation of the advisability for a spinal fusion. I hated being flipped on the Striker bed. It was terrifying and it hurt. So I made a deal with the doctors that I would sleep on my tummy at night and be on my back during the day so I could see what was going on. A year after my spinal fusions the pain became so awful that I couldn't do anything. It was terrible. My father took me every Monday to the clinic where they failed to find anything wrong. Finally, they decided to do exploratory surgery. They found that the bone they had transplanted in the first surgery had rotted away and that the spinal cord was exposed. I needed a third surgery! Had I done what had been prescribed, I could have really damaged myself. So one more operation and that was the end. After eight months or so in a body cast followed by physio, I was finally able to sit up and then resume my regular visits to the Constance Lethbridge Rehab Centre.

I was twenty before embarking on Grade 11 at Sir George Williams High School. Mr. Worrell who ran the bookstore (he too had had polio) persuaded me to go on to get my University degree as a mature student. The Town of Mount Royal Legion paid for my transportation. I got really involved in student activities and was even a member of the Garnet Key Society. They had to waive a rule about not sitting down while wearing the Garnet Key jacket! Later I was asked to correct papers for professors—really interesting. I was the second person in a wheelchair to attend the College. I loved Shakespeare, and was fortunate to have Neil Compton as one of my professors. He too was in a wheelchair having got polio as an adult the same year as I had, 1951. My four years at Sir George were the happiest of my life. I felt really useful and normal, with lots of friends who were real pals.

But society in general doesn't see us as normal human beings with feelings, hopes, and dreams. Children on the other hand are wonderful. They're so open with their questions. I think it's really important for children to be exposed to people with disabilities because they can accept the differences. On the surface, acceptance of people with handicaps might be better than in the past, but I wonder if it isn't just a facade.

I got married in 1970, and there were good times. But I was a battered wife, and like many others, I kept it to myself. The man tells you that you are no good, you're not worthy. So you believe it. And because marriage is the norm, it's hard to break out of a no-good situation. I kept thinking it was going to change. I was willing to forgive, willing to nurture a relationship hoping it was going to change, and so it had to get really bad before I finally realized it was never going to get any better. I had a normal sexual relationship with my husband. Let's get that out of the way, because people often wonder. A lot of the men who approached me romantically over the years had some sort of sexual hang-up. And I wouldn't know about these problems until I had formed a bond with them. That was hard. I came to realize that some of my pain today might come from the way I was treated in my earlier relationships. I just didn't seem to meet the right kind of men.

Troubles with pain and new weakness on my left side got me interested in Polio Quebec and the Polio Clinic at the Montreal Neurological Institute and Hospital. But my problem then turned out to be arthritis. I'm now coping with carpal tunnel syndrome stemming from my total dependence on my arms, hands, and wrists, and I'm doing whatever I can to avoid surgery and more months of lost independence. I have at last decided that the obvious first step in preserving my wrists is to take off weight, and my regime is working.

When my mother died, I had to learn to manage living alone. Getting in and out of bed, for instance isn't easy. It all takes a lot of time. First I have to put my stockings on because I can't move my legs without having something to grab onto. I wear petti-pants which are like a slip, so that I can slide, since I'm not strong enough to lift my bottom. I have to wear all this because otherwise my skin would get stuck on the leatherette of my wheelchair. And now that my hands don't work so well, it's harder. What's more, I have to have my back brace on because I can't sit up without it. This is my morning routine, but when in the middle of the night if there were to be a fire or an ammonia leak, for instance, everything would be all over by the time I'd be ready to move!

I'm having to get used to increasing tiredness, and during the heat waves this summer (1998) I started experiencing frightening breathing problems. Dr. Petrof, respirologist at the Royal Victoria Hospital, told me that most people can increase their breathing capacity when challenged, but that my reserve is very limited—at least 30 percent of normal. So I have to be very careful and go out only when the air is "good". Dr. Petrof has also recommended that I get flu shots as well as a pneumonia vaccine for protection. He has given me an inhaler just in case my problem is aggravated by allergies.

My biggest problem with this handicap has been the way people treat me. I try to laugh it off, but I must admit I don't like it when people talk to the person I am with about what I want, as if I didn't exist. I also regret not being given the opportunities to get ahead. I worked as a receptionist in the Students' Accounts Department at Sir George for seven years, but I was never promoted to the level of my abilities. I'm still angry about that. After my marriage broke up and I quit working, my home became a haven for children after school and on professional days as well as for the children whose parents had split up. These now-grown children keep in touch with me, which is wonderful. I did volunteer counseling work in a hospital and met people who made me realize my problems are small by comparison. I'm not the kind of person who dwells on what my life would have been like if… Instead of complaining, I just keep trying to figure out how to solve my problems.

I remember being approached by someone who wanted me to subscribe to a newspaper for people with handicaps. I was insulted that he thought I would need such a specialized paper, for in my eyes I was normal. We were pushed to be normal in the fifties and sixties, which I now feel was wrong. But later on I did get involved with handicap issues and managed to persuade the Town of Mount Royal to install an elevator in the Recreation Centre and the

City Hall in order to make its Council Meetings and recreational programs accessible. I am very proud of that. It took ten years of hard work.

During the winter months, loneliness has been a problem. Days can go by without my seeing a soul, and sometimes I feel sorry for myself. Occasionally around three or four in the afternoon, I often just start to cry for no reason. I don't have any family or relatives nearby and most of my good friends have left Montreal. I'd like to add that my neighbours are wonderful and I'm linked to the Town's telephone check called Daily Hello, but if anything were to go wrong there's nobody I could feel comfortable about calling. Scary at times.

Overall, I have gained from my experience with polio. Being in the hospital gave me my love and interest in people. I had so many opportunities to meet people of all ages. Something strange about nurses and doctors, though, is that they often talk about things as if one weren't there and couldn't understand anyway. But I was nosy, and I lapped it all up. I'm a determined person and I never accept that I can't do something until I have really tried.

My polio was hard on my parents financially as well as on Dad's career, but I never felt this until one day when I was mad about something, I said angrily to my father, "You never give me anything!" He replied, "The money I spent on your hospitalization could have taken us around the world three times." There were tears in his eyes. My parents had taken out accident insurance because I was a child who took lots of risks, especially on my bike, but this insurance did not cover polio. There was no Medicare in the 1950s. My dad died suddenly when I was twenty-one years old. This was difficult for both my Mum and me.

I used to love to travel and managed to cope long before accessible travel had even entered the vocabulary. They would carry me onto the plane. A friend would always accompany me unless I was going to visit someone who knew me well. I went to Venezuela, to Bermuda, to California, to Britain, and to Florida for Christmases. But those days are over because the late effects of polio are curbing my ability to travel. I'm still young and know that there are many more of life's adventures still ahead. I've more to learn, see and do, and best of all, new people and challenges to meet.

Daphne is now living in the Father Dowd residence where her vitality is appreciated.

The Will to Go On

Mona Arsenault

MY TWIN BROTHER and I were the youngest of five children. We contracted polio in 1952 at fourteen months of age. Of course I do not recall the original onset, but it was told to me many times. Early one morning my mother took us from our cribs and put us on the floor while she cleaned our room. As soon as she left me alone, I began to sniffle and cry. I had been walking for about two months, but that morning I just sat there, unable to move. My mom thought I had caught a cold from the window being left open overnight and called Dr. Mann, our family doctor. He came and after the examination sent both my brother and me immediately to the hospital. I was sent to the Montreal Children's Hospital, whereas my brother was sent to the Alexandra Pavilion, a hospital for contagious illnesses. His expression of polio was much worse, and the doctors were concerned about the severity of his lung problems. He had become instantly paralyzed from the face down, although I was only showing minor leg difficulties. Miraculously, Murray fully recovered within six months, whereas I remained unable to move my legs or walk.

Most of my early years were spent in and out of the Children's, rendering my four brothers as mysterious to me as I suppose I was to them.

My own first hospital memory is after the second operation when I was five. Groggily, I opened my eyes in the recovery room of the surgery ward where I spotted a little boy sitting on the end of my bed. I went back to sleep wondering whether it was just a dream. When I awoke a little while later, he was still there! I forced myself to stay awake this time and began to learn all about my renegade bed partner. He had been living in the recovery ward for over five years and needed constant intensive care. Daily the nurses carried him from bed to bed as they made their rounds. He was our "spot of sunshine", our "unexpected giggle".

The nurses were always checking our new casts and feeling our fingers and toes for circulation. Copying them, he would annoy the resting children whenever he had the chance. We were friends through difficult times. He spared my toes, that I can remember!

My fondest memories were of the student nurses. Their love and care of the youngsters made our lives a little easier. They were always compassionate and sensitive to the overwhelming number of children and managed to keep us happy. Seldom in those early years did I feel safe, but through them I experienced constant assurance of security and protection in an uncertain world.

I missed seeing my friends. My visitors were family members. After every operation, my mother would stay until I was stronger. My brothers would seldom visit, but my father, a taxi driver, popped in frequently. Sometimes he would show up at the end of his night shift and we would talk until he told me he got sleepy from his long hours of work. I would then tuck Dad into my bed, hop into my wheelchair, give him a kiss and a hug, and leave to seek out roommates until his nap was over.

The day before an operation became an event for Dad and me as the years passed. Instead of going to school, I would tour Montreal with him in his yellow-checkered cab. We would pick up fares, go to the mountain, and grab a lunch at Wilenski's Restaurant. We had some splendid times on these drives. Eventually, we would sign in at the hospital, often getting heck from the nurses for being so late. Dad had a knack for talking his way out of trouble and I must have developed my gift of the gab from him. Finally, our day would end when he tucked me into my hospital bed and told me not to worry.

My operations frequently took place during the Christmas break when the hospital was festive. I was often scared and anxious before an operation. Looking back, these hours were the most difficult part of any operation. One day, while I was nervously waiting for surgery, a nurse came in to ask me how I felt. I cried and told her how frightened I was. She disappeared into the corridor and returned moments later with wool and a hook. She began showing me how to crochet. Sitting up in bed, woozy from medication, I began flipping wool over the hook. I soon forgot my fears and have enjoyed arts and crafts ever since.

The problem with medical treatment and orthopedic surgery back then was that it was all trial-and-error. Orthopedic surgeons and their teams were handling mostly polio during the 1950s and 1960s. Their central theory was aimed at full recovery through "permanent corrective measures". So little was known about polio that nurses, physiotherapists, and doctors included me in their questions on what to do next. I was encouraged to tell them how I was doing or what I might need next. They discussed my ideas and we would come up with procedures and conclusions.

By the time I was thirteen years old, I had had surgery over twenty-five times. Following each one they told me, "After this problem has been corrected you will walk just like everyone else." They claimed these operations would make me better. "Now, this time you'll really see a difference." By the time I was fourteen I was finished with the Children's and wouldn't need any more operations. My physical co-ordination and dexterity had always been very good, however, the paralysis remained in my right leg and I had some residual weakness lingering in the left ankle. Although I used many types of braces between procedures, I could now walk without them. I occasionally relied on wooden crutches if I traveled far or stood for long periods. My new independence made me feel grown up. I put away all my childhood dolls, with their imaginary broken legs and makeshift casts.

My fourteenth was a year of many new beginnings. We moved to the suburbs and I attended a regular school, which was completely different from The School for Crippled Children. I remember the first year vividly, especially my first new "able" friend, Susan, and how we became inseparable. She would walk eight blocks to meet me at my house, and then go to school with me. Although I lived less than three blocks from school, it took us 45 minutes to get there because the doctors recommended to my mother that I walk without the use of crutches in order to strengthen my legs. Most of the time I used her arm for support. Sometimes we would sit on the curb resting until I could go on. She never complained about our long walks and I was very grateful for the company. My legs never did get stronger, but our friendship certainly did.

Summer camp was my best therapy. It opened my eyes to all the things I could do! The hospital world was a place where I did very little for myself, yet Camp Massawippi was magical. I soon realized most of the other campers were less capable than I was. Nowhere else in my life had I been one of the better walkers, yet here I was considered an able walker! My parents sent me treats all summer long, and visited on Family Days, bringing along my brothers and their friends. Amidst the games and the all-you-could-eat picnics, I had barrels of fun.

Within my family it was my mother who felt the impact of my polio the most. She often told me it was too hard for her to watch me fall wearing heavy leg braces or casts, and being forbidden to help. "She has to make it on her own," the doctors insisted. I managed, but it tore Mom up to see me struggle. I recall the many times we both cried about the unfairness of it all. Looking back, I am filled with a sense of gratitude that she did not dote over me. It was this very independence that enabled me to continue on my journey with the courage and the inner strength I have needed in tackling the things I have wanted to do.

Early in June 1967, at fifteen, after my final exam in high school, I took a city bus into town determined to find myself a summer job. By chance I found a job helping other teens find summer work. Canada Manpower had set up a program and needed volunteers to operate the phones. I was recruited and so began my ensuing non-profit career. At the end of my second work day, I got on a very crowded bus. No seats were available so I stood clinging to a post near the front, when all of a sudden the vehicle jerked to a stop and I toppled onto a stranger beside me. He was handsome. He began talking to me as I shyly listened. He told me his name was Marcy and other things about himself. Finally my stop arrived, I left to change busses and he followed me on to the next! He sat beside me even though there was plenty of room elsewhere. When my street arrived, I said good-bye, expecting him to remain seated, but he followed again. As I exited, so did he. Once outside, he asked if he could walk me home. It turned out he lived a few blocks from me. He invited himself into my house where we chatted and he asked me for a date for the following Friday. When I accepted, he kissed me! After he left I told Mom I was going to marry him. She told me I was foolish. After dating casually for several weeks I began having serious thoughts about Marcy. Out of the blue he broke off our friendship. I was devastated, and tried unsuccessfully to forget him. Marcy had been my first boyfriend and all my girl friends said I would soon meet someone else. It was not until the following spring that he called me. He called to tell me he was in the hospital undergoing an appendix operation and asked if I would visit him. I went and the rest is history. We have now been happily married for thirty-one years. Who says chance isn't lucky? He tells the story differently though. In his version, he says that I jumped on him and landed in his lap.

I have been fortunate enough to stay at home and dedicate my married life to raising our two loving, energetic sons Michael and Martin. In my spare time, I have pursued numerous interests within the volunteer community. My family has always been supportive of my unusual endeavours and for that I am deeply thankful.

Later in 1967 I became the youngest leader in Girl Guides. Guiding was an extraordinary experience that I enjoyed for over twenty years. I felt as if I was a part of the "regular" world. I organized groups of girls in the traditional Girl Guide way, until the day a desperate parent approached me with a question that was in need of an answer. She wondered if there was any group that her institutionalized mentally disabled daughter could join. I searched, yet there was none. Then I was inspired! I spent the next ten years leading Quebec's first Guide company for the intellectually impaired. This new group of women with special needs became an education for me, and I relished every moment. These activities further motivated me to undertake a college education and become a Special Care Technician, specializing in socio-cultural activities. I completed a thesis in community recreational planning where I focused on the concerns and integration of the public with able and less-able youth. This

Guide assembly needed a lot of support people to keep it functioning. I asked for volunteers through many free advertisements in the newspaper. I was generously rewarded.

That was when I met Michelle. She was eleven years old, and although she was disabled, her capabilities extended far beyond those of other members in the troop. She displayed a keen interest in the activities and for the first time, having spent most of her life as an outsider, she felt as if she belonged to something. Michelle remained with the group for many years, progressing up the ranks from Girl Guide to leader. Later, prompted by her dedicated father, I accepted Michelle as an academic student in my home. On her own she rode the bus for several hours to travel to our weekly meetings. I still tutor her to this day. I have helped others accomplish many great tasks, and have felt totally fulfilled. Through helping others, I no longer need in my life to be part of the "regular" world. I am part of the whole world.

In 1983, on my thirty-third birthday, my body went into shock. My muscles became painfully seized and immovable. I struggled in and out of reality as pain inexplicably jolted through my body. I was immediately admitted to the hospital. The next three days were the worst of my life. High fever, delirious dreams, irrational behavior, and depression accompanied this assault on my body. I was not in control of my life. No one was even sure what I was suffering from. I was carried home and spent a year looking for someone to tell me what was happening to my body. All the emergency room doctors, orthopedists, neurologists, sports medicine doctors, arthritic specialists, and psychiatrists did not understand, nor would they treat me. They told me to go home and tomorrow I would be fine. Naively trusting them, I would wake up each morning and inspect the sore spots to see if any pain had gone. It had not. Hoping made me anxious. I remembered my mother's words, "You'll be well when you grow up. All of us have problems in our lives. You have yours now while you're growing. Later you won't have any." It was extremely difficult to accept these physical changes in contrast to my previously active life. Through my husband's understanding, strength, and unlimited kindness I learned to ignore the professionals' unrealistic suggestions.

I read everything I could find about polio. When I came across an old book that described the original symptoms of acute polio, I noticed similarities. I believed I was suffering from polio again, though it was not diagnosed by any of the seventy-five physicians I sought out.

After a long year and a half, buoyed by courage and my family's strong belief in me, I ended up in the Aberhart Centre in Edmonton, Alberta, under Doctors Neil Brown and Rubin Feldman's expert polio care. I spent six weeks struggling back to health. The two ambitious doctors tried everything to get my body to cooperate. I was put through every imaginable test. Daily physiotherapy managed to revive me and enabled me to get out of bed for longer periods and walk again. These initial successes were not a solution, but the beginning of a long, arduous journey into a new life. The Aberhart Centre Polio Ward gave me invaluable memories of people who again changed my life. Most of them had been living there for many years and some had even been residents since the original polio had affected their lives.

Meeting people like Clayton May and Bill Karthaus made an indelible impression on me. Clayton May was a man among men. Amazingly, he could deliver energizing pep talks from his mechanical bed. He encouraged me to get on with my life and told me to get off my butt and start a polio support group in Quebec. His zeal for life must have come from his dwarfed size and the environment of contraptions needed to keep him alive. I believe his encouragement to others gave his life a greater meaning and purpose.

Bill Karthaus was also a resident of the Aberhart Centre and was more mobile than Clayton. On good days he used a manual wheelchair to get around. He seemed to be getting worse, yet it never held him back. He had experience with polio breathing difficulties, and thus felt the need to encourage patients on the Tuberculosis Ward. His many years in rocking beds or with oxygen masks made him an expert to the frightened new shut-ins. Every chance he had, he would put on a sterile gown and face mask, and talk for hours with a young child or elderly invalids in fear of their lives.

Darlene Stygels was a senior respiratory technologist working with long-term polio patients. She visited me often and helped me with my loneliness and insecure feelings about being sick and so far away from home. One day she asked me whether there was anything I wanted to see while in Western Canada. I replied, "I've never seen the Rockies." Without hesitation, she made arrangements with her intern husband to go on a trip to the mountains. I was overwhelmed. The voyage was longer than I expected, yet they were thrilled to drive the eight hours of twisted highway towards Banff National Park. It was a relief to be a tourist, not a patient!

A year later, back in Montreal, while undergoing more tests with the new polio specialist, Dr. Neil Cashman at the Montreal Neurological Institute, I became friends with a retired nurse who shared my room. She was from the Bahamas. One day she asked how far it was to St. Sauveur, a tourist town in the Laurentians she wanted to visit. Needless to say, my new friend and I had a lovely time the following sunny Sunday afternoon. I was fondly remembering my journey in the Rockies as my husband drove up to the Laurentian hills. Helping others heals.

While I was away, the Post-Polio Syndrome Association of Quebec

(L'Association québécoise pour le syndrome post-polio), now known as Polio Quebec, was born. Things were moving ahead. When I returned home from the Aberhart Centre the first thing I had to learn was to let others do for me what I had previously been able to do for them. It seemed impossible, I finally learned to ask for and accept the help that was willingly given. It was opportune that Polio Quebec had people with whom I could talk. They helped me understand what I believe to be my most difficult challenge, to accept my changed condition and take charge of myself. At this frightening stage in my adult life, I grabbed Polio Quebec by the horns and became its president. Post-polio and my affiliation with Polio Quebec enabled me to meet the family I never knew I longed for. Shared history and a sense of belonging are very comforting. Through this second disability, I have gained unique friendships and insights. I thank them for listening when I needed to be listened to, for believing in me when I could not, and teaching me to believe in myself.

My condition did stabilize over the next ten years, and at fifty, I am beginning to notice other changes. I realize now that muscles which were previously unaffected, are slowly becoming weaker. These changes have motivated me to tighten control over my body and figure out new inventive ways to keep it in shape. I now listen carefully to what my body tells me, and somehow together my body and I will overcome the challenges we face. I strongly believe it has been my positive attitude that has enabled me to cope with the curves I have been thrown. I will not pretend that it has been easy to escape negativity's grasp, but the realization of the importance of the Now may be the mightiest armour one can have.

The Now is all I have. "Back then" or "later on" have no power here. So seize it, control it, understand it, and most of all, revel in it, for it is ours to wield. I do, and therein lies my strength.

I Am More than My Polio

HELEN D'ORAZIO

I WAS BORN IN MONTREAL on August 30, 1952. At two months of age, when my mother was bathing me she lifted my arm to wash it and she noticed it just seemed to fall back down. She was told I had polio. Mom remembers I had just received a needle three days earlier at the hospital for a vaccination, which I assume, was for D.P.T. (diphtheria, tetanus, and whooping cough). She seemed to think maybe the needle was dirty and that's how I must have gotten polio. No one ever mentioned if I was hospitalized at the time, what tests were done, or if I was isolated from others. It was never talked about and somehow I think I felt I wasn't supposed to ask.

Recently I had the opportunity to view my chart at the Montreal Children's Hospital. I had been hospitalized for five days where diagnostic tests were done to determine if I indeed had polio. My left arm was completely paralyzed. I had weakness in my right leg as well as some weakness in the left side of my face. A lumbar puncture was done where a sample of the cerebrospinal fluid is taken to determine if the poliovirus is present. It was negative. The doctors thought that maybe it was a brain lesion, which could explain the facial weakness but not the paralysis. I was sent home and had many physiotherapy treatments. As time went on they felt my symptoms were more compatible with polio.

My early recollections of polio come from when I started school. There was no kindergarten back then. I started grade one at six years old and that was also the year of my first surgery. I remember my left arm was completely paralyzed at the time. I could swing it all around by pushing it with my right arm. It seemed to be something I was proud of.

I don't remember much of the first two hospitalizations. I do remember the smell of Ivory soap at bath time and the noise of the dishes and the smell of the food in the kitchen and the melamine dishes I ate out of. The only story my mother would tell me on more than one occasion was of me crying after she visited me in the hospital. She found it hard to leave. I got to walk to the playroom while others with legs in traction were wheeled in with their beds. I remember watching movies. I will never forget the treatment room. That's where they would take you early in the morning to prepare you for surgery. I would get shaved and washed with an antiseptic soap and returned to my bed to wait for the operating room stretcher.

Dr. Farfan was my orthopedic surgeon. His goal was to make my arm as functional as possible. When I was seven years old he did tendon transfers of the wrist and left thumb. I could now bring my thumb to touch my other fingers, which I couldn't do before. I could also bend my wrist. Dr. Farfan seemed pleased. I suppose if he was pleased then I should be too, although the rest of my arm was still paralyzed.

Six months later I received a tendon transfer of the elbow. Now I could bring my hand up to my shoulder without assistance but when I tried to straighten my arm I couldn't. It seemed my arm was always sticking out. I was embarrassed and as I was getting older my body was growing and getting bigger but my left arm was staying small and I couldn't straighten it.

At fifteen I had another surgery, a fusion of the shoulder. A body cast with my left arm supported in mid-air had been molded on to me before surgery and allowed to dry for two days. It was then split on the right side, removed and reapplied in the operating room. The day before I was discharged, a new body cast was applied with the help of attendants holding my arm in position. This cast was part of me for three months. I was an adolescent in Grade 10 and too embarrassed to go to school looking like this. My sister brought my homework from school and I spent much of my time studying and subsequently managed to pass my school year. After much physiotherapy I was now able to move my shoulder a little and lift my arm about three inches in all directions. Again the doctors were pleased with my functioning shoulder. I could hold up to four pounds in my hand for a short period of time. I remember becoming even more self-conscious at the time because now my shoulder was no longer rounded and smooth. The fusion had caused a bone to stick out.

I recall many visits to physiotherapy and the orthopedic clinic to see Dr. Farfan. It was a familiar routine. My mom and I would enter the hospital on Dorchester Boulevard. We would register and then I would get a carton of chocolate milk at the mini-snack bar. The orthopedic clinic was on the second floor. Our appointment was always at one o'clock and so was everyone else's. We had to sit on hard benches in the waiting room that reminded me of church pews. When my name was called, which would often be around three o'clock, I would go into the examination room, be told to undress to my underwear and wait for the doctor, his residents, and interns. Dr. Farfan would touch my arm, ask me to move my fingers, bend my elbow, and lift my shoulder. He was showing me off to the other doctors. Then he would ask me to walk back and forth. Why? I didn't know. After seeing my chart I learned that my right leg was a little shorter than the left, and this was when I was twelve years old. I also had a mild dorsal scoliosis. I continued being followed by Dr. Farfan until I was eighteen years old at which point I was considered an adult and no longer needed to be seen at a children's hospital. Everything that could be done to make my arm as functional as possible had been done.

I was the third of six children, four girls and two boys. My mother was not only busy with a daughter who had polio; there was my oldest sister Pauline, who was mentally retarded, who she had to deal with. Pauline was a handful for my parents, especially my mother because my father was often on shift work. When he worked nights, he had to sleep during the day and Mom would always tell us not to make so much noise, because Dad was trying to sleep. He also worked many evenings so Mom would be alone with the six of us. My mother's brother also lived with us. He used a hearing aid most of the time because of deafness caused during the war. He was also a handful at times because he needed to be hospitalized a few times for a nervous condition. We were nine people living in a three-bedroom house. Pauline often had temper tantrums and would certainly very often get her way just to keep the peace. Whenever we were upset over her rearranging our belongings in our room or taking something of ours, we were told, "You know what she's like. She's sick, just let her be." If one of us would misbehave, we were told, "You have a head on your shoulders, you're not sick like your sister. You should know better."

Mom's nickname was "Speedy Gonzales" because she would do so much and so fast. We never really learned to cook because it was quicker for Mom to do it all herself. I know Mom must have felt burdened with six children, one who was mentally retarded, one with polio, and also a "shell-shocked" brother. I felt I was one of her burdens, so I made sure I would do everything expected of me to make her life a little easier. I was a good girl. There was something wrong with me just like there was something wrong with my sister Pauline. I worried that people would think of me the same way that they thought of Pauline.

As a child I was overprotected. I remember being told, "Be careful. Can you do that with your little arm?" I liked sports; I played hopscotch and enjoyed skipping rope. I liked gymnastics. I wanted to be on the basketball team in high school but the gym teacher wouldn't let me because she was afraid I would get hurt. I didn't like people telling me I couldn't do something.

Growing up I was always very self-conscious about my body, even though the polio had only affected my left arm. It was never really talked about in the family. I had it. Everyone knew and that was it. Whatever treatments, surgeries, and physical attention were needed, were taken care of.

I felt I was on my own to deal with my feelings about having polio. I felt different. There was something wrong with me because my arms were not the same length or the same size. I was a shy child, always worrying what other people thought of me. I was scared that if they knew I had polio, I wasn't perfect and they wouldn't like me. I wasn't all that surprised when I saw a notation in my chart that read "Mother feels Helen is perfect except for her arm." I tried very hard to be liked at home and at school. I was able to hide my deformed arm most of the time. I either wore long sleeved blouses to hide my arm or short-sleeved T-shirts that would hide my bony shoulder, but never sleeveless tops! If I talked to someone I would sometimes stand behind a doorway so that my left arm was out of view. People would see my legs, my body, and only my right arm. That way I felt on even ground with other people. Whenever I was in a picture with at least two people, I would position myself so that my left arm would be behind someone. It almost became an obsession with me to hide my arm. If I couldn't see my arm then maybe others couldn't see it either. With friends and family this feeling of wanting to hide my arm wasn't as strong as when I met people for the first time.

I would think, if I were nice and friendly toward them, they would probably like me. I worried they would change their minds if and when they ever found out I had polio.

Would they pity me? I always worried that they might not like me or that I wasn't good enough for them.

It was during my last hospital stay that I realized I wanted to be a nurse. The nurses were always so nice and friendly. They seemed to know a lot and they always had an answer. They were good people and the patients liked what they did for them. That was what I was going to become. I was going to be SOMEBODY.

I remember overhearing a relative ask Mom once how I was doing with the polio. She answered, "Well, I guess she's doing fine because she never talks about it." I don't really know how my polio affected my brothers and sisters because we rarely talked about it and we still don't. It's not easy for me to bring up the subject although it's something I am presently working on.

I keep in touch with a few friends that I've had since childhood. Carmela and Lucy were very surprised to hear that it was on my mind constantly as a child. They never felt it was an issue. Carmela said she was amazed at how well I could catch the ball when we played dodge ball at school. They both knew I had polio. They thought I just went on with my life. They liked me because we were friends.

I became good friends with Mary in Grade 10 after my last surgery. She always reminded me that if I couldn't do one thing there was always something else I could do. Whenever I put myself down she would always find a way of picking me up by finding something good in me.

I've been married twenty-six years now and have two children. Anthony is twenty-three and Rosanne is twenty. I remember thinking no one would want to marry me because I wasn't perfect but my husband Mario persevered. He didn't see me as disabled. Our love and trust has grown deeper over the years. This past summer I really enjoyed our camping vacation throughout the Gaspé coast.

I found it physically difficult at times when my children were little. I always envied the parents who could hold their baby in one arm and do something with the other arm like answer the phone or plug in the kettle or get milk from the fridge or even bend to pick up a pacifier that had fallen. As the children got older they just knew I had a weaker arm and I managed somehow with the other arm.

I worked as a nurse at the Montreal General Hospital for twenty-six years, which is something I am very proud of. I'm sure my previous hospital experience as a patient helped me become a better nurse because I could identify with my patients' needs. I worked full-time in orthopedics and recovery room for five years until I had Anthony. Since then I worked part time on the float team never knowing until I arrived at work if I would be assigned to Emergency, Intensive Care, or a General Floor. I must admit I enjoyed working in the Coronary Care Unit the most because of the camaraderie of the nurses. I truly enjoyed helping people and got so much satisfaction and acceptance in return. The workload was a little less physically demanding there than on other floors. I managed to do with one strong arm what others did with two good ones.

I did pull a ligament in my lower back fifteen years ago and I was unable to work for six months. This was the first time I had ever heard the word "post-polio syndrome" spoken to me by the staff doctor. I remember saying to myself, "What in heaven's name is she talking about? I just hurt my back lifting a patient! My polio is history!" When I returned to work, I was always very cautious of reinjuring my back. I decreased my number of shifts from twelve to eight in six weeks. I worked evenings so the children wouldn't be with a babysitter for long. I prepared supper before leaving for work. I put in a full day at home. By the time I left for work I was already tired. My eight-hour work shift was always so busy there was no time to relax. I would arrive home exhausted and feel tired for two more days.

A few years later I pulled my back again and this time I saw a chiropractor who told me my right leg was a little shorter than the left. I always had a high arch on my right foot that I felt was related to the polio. It had never caused any problems. It was at this time I recalled a staff doctor mentioning post-polio syndrome. This prompted me to ask my family doctor to refer me to the post-polio clinic. If my leg problem was related to my polio I wanted to see someone who was familiar in this area. I was now thirty-nine years old and had seen no polio specialist since I was eighteen.

I met with Dr. Trojan who ran the post-polio clinic at the Montreal Neurological Institute. She examined me and prescribed orthotics, specially molded insoles that help rebalance the foot. X-Rays to determine any leg length discrepancy showed my right leg was shorter by 0.8 centimetres. I was prescribed an elevation for my shoe. She also discussed symptoms of post-polio syndrome, which I ignored because I was feeling fine. At this time I was doing low impact aerobics three times a week and keeping up quite well. I enjoyed cross-country skiing and even took lessons in downhill skiing, although I could never get past the beginner level. At this late age I had learned how to swim which was something I was so determined to do and so proud of. At one point I was swimming forty laps in one hour.

Over the years I was having more difficulty keeping up with the intensity of the aerobic classes. I decreased to two days of aerobics and one day of aqua-fit and eventually only did aqua-fit. It seemed less tiring than aerobics although I remember feeling burning in my thighs even in the water. I slowed my pace rather than try to keep up with everyone else.

After my first consultation with Dr. Trojan I continued working one day a week. I would often feel a burning sensation and aching in my upper back and shoulder of the right arm at work that would sometimes last a couple of days. This was not the arm that had the polio involvement, or so I thought. I kept telling myself this was getting physically harder for me but I just wanted to keep working until I reached twenty-five years service. I didn't want to stop working. What would I do? My solution would have to wait.

During the unforgettable ice storm of 1998 in Quebec, my house burned down due to a defective installation of the fireplace. Our cat perished in the fire. We lost everything. We were left with the clothes on our backs. I took a leave of absence from work for one year in order to oversee the rebuilding of the house, do the inventory for the insurance company, and take care of my husband and children. I also did most of the shopping for clothes and furnishings for the house. It seemed to be an endless task. By the time all this was over ten months had gone by. I could finally start thinking about myself again. That's when I became aware of discomfort in my neck and shoulders. Massages that usually helped were now aggravating the condition. I foolishly returned to work in January, exactly one year after the fire. After three shifts I realized something must be wrong. Nothing seemed to help the pain, which was worsening. I finally saw a doctor, having first consulted an osteopath and a physiotherapist. By March 1999 the results of my scans were in. I had severe spinal stenosis as well as a cervical herniated disc. I was in pain twenty-four hours a day. Nothing relieved the pain for more than an hour. I tried acupuncture. I was getting depressed from being in constant pain. Because I believed this problem must be related to the polio, I asked Dr. Trojan to refer me to a specialist. I finally saw Dr. Pokrupa in July and had surgery in October, a year after my symptoms started. It's been a long and difficult rehabilitation process. If I didn't believe I had post-polio syndrome before the surgery, I certainly do so now. My neck and shoulder muscles were so weak I had to wear one of those hard stiff neck collars for six months just to help keep my head up and I was constantly tired.

I had an electromyography that showed the polio involvement was more widespread than previously thought. All four limbs were affected, not just the left arm I had always grown up believing. No wonder my right arm was starting to let me down. The strength that I could always depend on and the endurance just weren't there anymore. My legs were feeling the effects as well. Now, I wear a splint on the right foot for a foot drop that seems to have been slowly getting worse over the years. My quadriceps are weaker and my legs tire faster. I take shorter walks.

It's been three years now and I'm still learning to manage my energy level. Most days I either sleep in the afternoon or rest on and off. I'm learning to pace myself. When I sit, I try to find a chair with a high back or I try to lean against a wall if I can. I try to slow down or stop when I get tired. I actually notice that listening to my body makes a difference. Some days I still overdo it.

I'm on disability insurance now. Even though I wasn't working full time I miss feeling useful because of what I could do as a nurse. My challenge now is not dwelling on what I can't do but finding new value in what I can do. I am very grateful that I can walk, I can drive, and I can socialize. I think because I've learned to listen to my body better, I can now take part in an aqua arthritis program. It feels great to be back in the water. My body still reminds me that it needs to be listened to constantly.

I've also joined Toastmaster's which is an organization that helps its members gain more confidence by practicing public speaking, which is something I've always wanted to do.

If anything positive came from my having polio, it would be my drive to succeed despite my polio. I always wished I had never had polio because then I would have felt more normal. I now question whether my polio was the only reason I tried so hard to please other people so they could like me.

I've become more active in the Polio Quebec Association. Growing up I had never met anyone with polio, and now I feel there are people like me out there. I feel less alone and so much more connected as I get to know these new friends. I am looking forward to getting to know some of them better.

I'm finding it a little less difficult asking for help now. I'm realizing that the most important person that needs to like me is myself, and the rest will just have to fall into place.

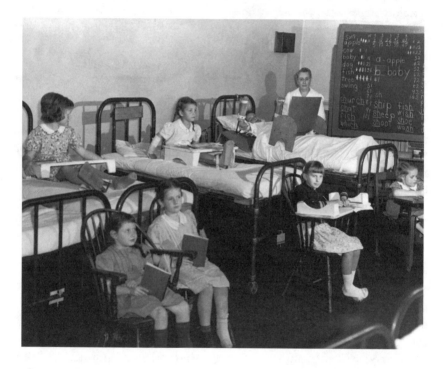

A class for young polio patients at Sick Kids.
The Hospital for Sick Children (Toronto), Hospital Archives.

Very Glad to Be Alive

Eileen Gagnon

It was in the Gaspé, July 1953, that polio struck me and my family. I was two years and eight months old. It affected my pelvis and my legs and kept me from walking for a good seven months. It was thought that my brother also had a mild case because he had a fever and a stiff neck. The doctor recommended giving him an enema. Whatever the reason, he recovered without any polio symptoms. I was hospitalized for a month in the Gaspé area, followed by six months in Ste. Justine, a Montreal children's hospital full of polios. The following September I had to be hospitalized again and I remember being left there by my mother. To get away without a scene, she told me she had forgotten her gloves at home. But she didn't return.

My memories about those days are a bit confused, but I remember women coming to visit me. They must have been my father's sisters. They brought me presents.

When I returned home I had physio once a week for years. Madame Edpart would come and put me through my exercises in our living room. Nice as she was, I hated every minute of my time with her. I started school late because the first year was delayed by my frequent bouts with bronchitis caused by muscular weakness in my chest. Infections were so common that I had to return to the hospital where I was put in an oxygen tent. I had lots of operations and needed a brace for a while. By shortening a muscle in my hip, however, I was able to discard the brace, and I fell less often. While at university I had another operation, and it was excruciatingly painful. Nobody could understand why it was so sore. They wanted to open me up again to find out what the problem was. I was literally paralyzed by the pain. I couldn't do a thing. My mother would try to comfort me. She felt suffering had to be endured, that we have no power over our lives. For her, life was full of suffering, a cross that had to be borne. But I refused to be a victim. The only solution it seemed at the time was to end my life.

Aged 27, I took an overdose of 222s, and that night I was finally at peace with myself. If there is 'something' elsewhere, that was where I was going. In the middle of the night I was as sick as a dog, threw up all the pills, and slept soundly. When I woke up the next morning, I was fine and very glad to be alive. Somehow I felt free. Life was miraculously no longer a burden. I had liberated myself from my Catholic upbringing, one which considers suicide a sin and life a burden that has to be lived even when it is unbearable. Don't get me wrong—life hasn't been a bed of roses, but when I get depressed I now know that I have a choice. I ask myself: "Do I still want to live?" and since the answer is still "Yes", I rally my strength and live fully.

When I was young I didn't like getting undressed in front of the doctors and residents. I felt all alone, being examined like an object, for we polio kids were like guinea pigs. I have done my share of being used as a teaching tool and I won't take it any more, and I don't!

I calculate that I have spent two and a half to three years on my back. Have these long hours of immobility made me more contemplative than someone who hasn't experienced all these physical and emotional challenges? Am I more able to look deeper at life and reflect before rushing into action? When you are prone on your back, there's little else to do but think, being in no mood to read. Normally I love to read. Was this passive or contemplative behaviour? To sum it all up, polio taught me perseverance.

Knowing what I do now, I have no idea whether I would make the same decisions about managing my handicap if I had to do it all over again. I find orthopedic surgery very violent. I question whether Mézière treatment or osteopathy would have been a viable alternative. After all, I didn't have a severe back problem to begin with. One doctor in particular treated just a part of me, failing to take my whole body into account. As a result, he operated on my knee, reinforcing the muscle in front, weakening the two muscles behind my knee. He was far too quick to use the knife. As a result, I can no longer bend this knee without helping it. So when I walk, my leg is stiff and I have to rotate to move forward. That happened in 1973. It throws me off balance, and I have to walk with a cane. The real problem was that my back was getting worse, and the operation hadn't dealt with that problem.

Polio had a terrible impact on my childhood. It separated me from my brothers and sisters. My mother kept me apart. She over-protected and spoiled me. I think being spoiled is one of childhood's worst handicaps and gets in the way of normal socializing. But I don't blame my mother. She was doing what she believed to be best. I would have been better off had she put me in a home with other children where I could have learned from the start to fend for myself.

I went to a regular school, but even there I felt the children overprotected me. I was accepted more as a cute kid who needed help than for whom I was. Somehow, it felt unreal.

Medical expenses were a curse. We were poor, charity cases. My mother had to cope with social workers and the like who weren't always polite to her. My brothers and sisters didn't experience this humiliation because they didn't have to deal with that outside world that my polio thrust my mother and me into.

I have some good memories of my time in Ste. Justine Hospital, particularly about the student nurses. I remember their blue, pink, and striped uniforms, their aprons and caps, and the children in embroidered jackets. Those doctors, Dr. Pierre Labelle in particular, were like good daddies when I was young, just as the nurses were like good mommies. Of course, there were exceptions.

My mother wanted to send me to Victor Doré School for children with handicaps, but I didn't want to go, even though my childhood was marked by the feeling of being on the sidelines of a normal world. Paradoxically I might have been able to have a better image of myself if I had known other children who were handicapped with whom I could relate to or identify with.

All of this must have been very difficult for my family, for my mother in particular. Although she would deny it, having a female child who was handicapped left its mark on her as a woman. My sister, for instance, always seemed to be seeking out illness to make herself interesting. My brother who was a year younger was very quiet. He didn't bother any one. But my mother didn't let my brothers and sisters act normally with me. She prevented, even prohibited, any aggressivity. A positive result of all this, I think, is that our shared experience with my handicap made my family members sensitive and compassionate.

At the age of sixteen I realized I needed help and found a psychologist by looking in the Yellow Pages. It cost me an exorbitant $15 an hour back then which I paid with money earned babysitting. It was worth it.

I sometimes imagine myself running and being without the discomfort of my body, and I find that I envy those who are able to walk straight, who can easily put one foot in front of the other without having to plan each step. This feeling makes me sad. Nonetheless, I tolerate my handicap and learned that there's more to life than being like everyone else. It is more important to feel free and in control of one's destiny. When I listen to the frustrations of older people who have to deal with the limitations of aging, I realize that this is what I have been doing all my life. Does this make me better prepared for the aging process? I could have done without it so young!

If I had to start my life over again I would ask my mother to let me work things out with other children on my own. Her feelings of pity and discomfort towards my handicap, even though she didn't show it overtly, affected me. She was always trying to protect me and to anticipate what might be best for me. It seems that when one is handicapped, people are less attracted to you; I felt this particularly during my adolescent years. On weekends, for instance, my friends would go out together, but they wouldn't include me. This marked me. As an adult, I am able to defend myself better. Now I realize that those who can't see beyond my disability are really more handicapped than I am. They need glasses!

As for my relationship towards men, that is the most difficult chapter of my life. The same factors that came into play during my childhood figured in my socializing with men. It wasn't easy. My mother held my sister in great esteem and this really got to me, that is, feeling on the sidelines of social life and in addition, being set apart from the rest of the family by my mother. My face might have been beautiful, I was even intellectual, but that wasn't enough. Boys took to my sister. They didn't seem to notice me. It still troubles me. If my mother had only been able to focus on other values besides appearances, and to appreciate me for whom I was, I would have had more self-confidence. I was always frightened men would choose me because they couldn't have anyone else. I wondered why they were interested in me. I just didn't believe in myself. I didn't have the feeling of being important. Could it be that men find it difficult to really care for a woman who is handicapped? Do they look for normalcy to begin with? I must admit, there were some men who weren't even aware of my being handicapped. They could see beyond it and this helped me begin to overcome my feeling of rejection. If as a child you are constantly told you can't do things or go places because you are handicapped, it leaves a lasting impression—and one that I have worked to overcome.

I am now dealing with a few post-polio symptoms such as fatigue. My joints are less supple, I'm much weaker, but fortunately my body has inherited a good resistance to these problems. My recent surgery was really tough, but it hasn't changed things. It reinforced what had been done in the past and got rid of my back pain. But yes, I still have pain in my joints, my legs feel heavy and my neck is stiff. An osteopath is working on my neck problem. Alternative medicines, such as Mézière, osteopathy, and shiatsu have been a great help to me over the years. In addition, I swim twice a week and am greatly helped by an Aqua Jogger vest which keeps me buoyant while I exercise different parts of my body. I avoid medication unless absolutely necessary. It is a last resort for me because I'm scared there may be side effects. Sometimes they are worse than the cure. I live as naturally as possible. If I can't sleep, I do relaxation exercises.

If you were to tell me today, "Eileen, you have a choice of having your polio taken from you along with all that you have learned as a result of having had it," I would be upset. Although I would prefer not to have had polio, I think I gained a lot from the experience. I have no idea what life would have been like without it, but I think there is a sensitivity and a depth to my personality that wouldn't be there without having gone through what I did. I probably would have been quite superficial. Because I couldn't do what everyone else was doing, I read a lot. I was able to help the younger members of my family. I think I influenced them quite a bit. I was helped by psychotherapy—it was like a second education. I was sixteen when I first recognized the need for this kind of support, but I only went a few times because I didn't have much money. Then I continued when I was nineteen. It gave me a feeling of being the oldest in the family, even though I wasn't. I felt like the leader. Having an opportunity to reflect upon my handicap and come to terms with it positively changed how I felt about myself, irrespective of my handicap. No longer were the opinions of others reflected in my self-image.

My brothers didn't hesitate to let me know that they found me pugnacious and adventurous. The fact that I would dare to hitchhike impressed them, as did the fact that I succeeded in my studies and gained professional status. Polio played its part in my career choice and how I carry it through. It made me more sensitive to the profound suffering of others and to each person's unique ability to pull out of it with whatever means he or she has. My tactics are confrontational and quite creative. I also have a well developed intuitive sense which doubtless comes from having had long periods of being virtually alone in the hospital surrounded by strangers and unable to do much more than observe and reflect.

We Get from Life What We Give to It

JIMMY COTTER

I FELT ILL ON A SATURDAY in the autumn of 1953, aged twenty. I had a headache that I believed to be a hangover. By Sunday I was perspiring with fever. My doctor insisted I go for a lumbar puncture, and sure enough, Dr. Monroe Bourne diagnosed me with polio. I was taken to the Alexandra Pavilion that afternoon where I was quarantined for two weeks. Three days after being admitted, I was placed in an iron lung where I remained for nine weeks. It looked like a big old-fashioned washing machine. Except for my head, my whole body was inside with the air pressure breathing for me. There were portholes through which the nurse could take care of my hygiene and wash me. Soft felt around these portholes stopped air from escaping. When they had to work on my entire body, they put a big plastic bubble over my head. They could then open the respirator and slide me out on a stretcher and work on me without interfering with the air pressure.

My first two weeks in the iron lung were tormented by nightmares; I was cutting my throat, or stabbing myself with scissors, and I remember the panic when under the plastic bubble I wasn't getting enough oxygen. The nurses thought it was my just being scared, but it turned out to be a malfunction. Needless to say, it sort of destroyed my confidence in that plastic bubble. But at the Alexandra there were always nurses nearby, so if a respirator malfunctioned or there was a power outage, they would swing into action with a hand pump.

I'm still in touch with the wonderful head nurse, Laleila (Jenny) Wren. The Alexandra was a training institution; so every six weeks we would have a new batch of nurses from all the hospitals. They were kept on their toes by Nurse Wren, which resulted in excellent care. Weaning me from the iron lung took about four weeks on a chest respirator, a sort of shield like a baseball umpire's chest protector which I needed less and less over that period. From the Alexandra I was sent to the Western (Montreal General) until June 15. My ability to walk came back slowly by Christmas. My left leg regained almost normal strength, but my right leg can't bear weight when my knee is bent. I was hospitalized for a total of eight months.

Although my polio was diagnosed in Montreal, I'm not sure where it came from. I used to swim in many of the Laurentian lakes around Lac Marois. I had three groups of friends—my own personal group, the group that I worked with, and a group on the Lakeshore that I played football with. I was the only one in all these three groups that came down with polio. How do you explain that? I didn't think too much of my diagnosis because about eight years previously I had a friend who had had polio, and it was hardly noticeable. I'd never known anyone who had it more severely, so of course I thought I would soon be out of the hospital, take a holiday and then go back to work at the bank after Christmas.

I was a client of the Institut de Réadaptation from 1954 to about 1956, off and on, under Dr. Mongeau. They sent me to New York, to the Institute of Physical Medicine and Rehabilitation—Howard Rusk's Institute, part of the Bellevue Medical Center. They tried to make a brace for me here in Quebec. It was the March of Dimes back then that made it possible for me to spend nine weeks in New York where a unique brace was made, by trial and error, guided by the occupational therapist. It had a cable attached to the forearm that went up my sleeve, down my back anchored to a belt round my waist. The cable went down my pant leg to a robin's-egg-like thing attached to my shoe, like a fishing reel with a brake on it—a bar—and when I stepped on the bar, the fishing reel wound up and locked, so when I straightened my leg, it pulled on the cable and lifted my arm. It was how I was able to hold a pen or a pencil, so I could write, just by the movement of my body, by holding my arm at the desk level, and when I wanted to type I just took a pencil without an end on it and typed as you would with one finger. I could only master a limited speed. Dr. Underecker was the resident in charge of my file.

After a year, they wanted me back in New York to complete the hand-piece at Bellevue. And what a good recreational program they had, too—professional baseball games, football games, basketball, an opening at Radio City Music Hall, a championship boxing match. There were always a couple of station wagons at our disposal so that on weekends we could take off.

The man who made the brace was a paraquad, having been in a terrific car accident. However, he was a perfectionist. His, or should I now say my brace is featured in a rehab textbook, and a video has been made about it for teaching purposes. I'd only wear the brace for work. It would take ten to fifteen minutes to get me strapped into it. I don't wear it any more, though, but it enabled me to work all those years. When I had mastered it with the help of the Rehab in Montreal, they offered me a part-time job. For six years I worked half days. Then the new Institute was built and I accepted a full-time position. I was there for thirty-nine years, until January 1995 when I got pneumonia.

My pleasant memories of the hospital are those of the nurses. We were all about the same age, which made it a lot more pleasant. We talked about the same things, the same jokes. Now that I'm in a nursing home—I'm the baby here at The Bayview—I'm about the same age as many of the nurses. Makes me think of all those young nurses way back in the 1950s who were my age. What a difference it made to my hospital life.

I lifted weights. I figured it was a good thing to do, but it certainly didn't strengthen my leg. I'd learned long ago to do crossword puzzles at night without my brace, so that is now how I write.

My friends all stuck by me and still visit. If I had stayed home after my pneumonia, I would have been very much alone with just a CLSC nurse visiting twice a day. That's why I wanted to be in this nursing home—near them. It's like being in a resort—nice people and a great view overlooking Lake St. Louis. Réné Dallaire invited me out sailing last summer in Ken Francis' program, but the wind was very strong that day, so I stayed on shore, having been warned to avoid catching cold.

Paying expenses was difficult. Dad died in 1951 and my mother was just getting the old age pension. My sister and three brothers were no longer in Montreal. My mother was getting ready to sit back and enjoy life, and—Bang!—I got sick. She was the one who took care of me from 1953 into the 1970s when her health failed and we had to get people to come in. She died in 1976.

The top third of my lung didn't come back after my polio. In 1995 I got pneumonia. Tubes were thrust down my throat. They performed a tracheotomy and sent me to the Montreal Chest Hospital to recuperate. I developed sleep apnea, so was prescribed a BiPap machine. It breathes with me and should I stop breathing, after ten seconds it will pump air into me, and if I don't start after nineteen seconds, an alarm goes off and a nurse will rush in to wake me up. Tests showed that not only do I have a lung functioning at two-thirds capacity, but also that one side of my diaphragm is completely shot. The doctors determined that there was nothing that could be done surgically to mend the damage, so that is why I now have to use the BiPap to sleep. Twice a week it needs sterilizing, and the inhalation therapist comes to inspect it from time to time. My friends have been wonderful.

I lived in Montreal's Côte-des-Neiges district, and when I needed to be placed in a caring environment, they wanted to place me in that area. But my family was miles away, and my friends were on the Lakeshore. So eventually, with a social worker's help, I got transferred to Bayview in Dorval, and it's wonderful.

When I realized I was going to have to give up my way of life after the pneumonia, I soon realized that being in a place like the Bayview was so much more pleasant than being by myself at home, waiting for the caregiver. The downside of my new weakness is that I can't go anywhere without lugging this BiPap equipment with me, which I am unable to do.

Looking back, I've met a lot of new people and made new friends. I have learned that I get from life what I invest in it. Everybody is dealt a hand, and you just have to cope with it as best you can by remembering the positives and letting the negatives fall by the wayside.

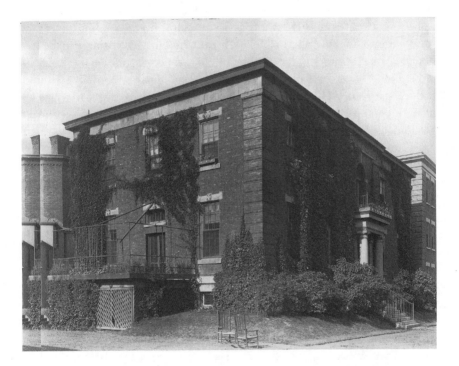

Alexandra Hospital, Pointe St. Charles, 1920.
Notman Historical Archives.

Unless He Remembers to Take a Breath, He Can't

GARY MCPHERSON

IN 1955, AT THE AGE OF NINE, Gary Mcpherson contracted polio, and since then he has lived with only limited movement of one hand and one leg. When not using a ventilator, his breathing is conscious, not autonomic, and that means unless he remembers to take a breath, he can't. Over the years he has developed a profound understanding of life and people, and he uses this gift to help others overcome obstacles. This book would not be complete without including his story. His example of overcoming, or perhaps disregarding what to some people would seem to be insurmountable obstacles, he does with wit, wisdom, charm, and sheer willpower.

From his website (www.garymcpherson.com) one learns that after his fortieth birthday he decided to take his health into his own hands. Despite his severe quadriplegia, he moved away from the medical institutions that he had called home for thirty-four years, from October 1955 to October 1989. It was only then that he moved into his own home with his new wife Valerie. They now have two treasured children, Keiko and Jamie. Gary's experience with polio was always a challenge. He faced many life-threatening occasions because polio had paralyzed most of his chest and abdominal muscles. He could not breathe on his own and required a ventilator twenty-four hours a day.

In order to ease the flow of air to his lungs, doctors performed a tracheotomy that might have helped Gary's breathing, but it resulted in his experiencing numerous serious infections. One night in 1957, Gary woke up to find that his tracheal tube had come out of his neck and the opening had closed over to the point that the doctors could not put it back in without performing a surgical procedure. At this point he made the brave decision to do without the tracheal tube. In 1962 Gary learned glossopharyngeal breathing (commonly called "frog" breathing)—a red-letter achievement that would eventually allow him freedom from his ventilator during the day and enable him to participate in many community activities.

Polio had a major impact on his entire family. Since there was no help for Gary in the Yukon where they lived, his family moved down to Edmonton to be near him. His dad found work, but at a much lower salary than what he was earning in the Yukon. The financial challenges eventually forced his mother back to work outside the home. By this time Gary had three siblings, including his seven-year-old sister who missed him dreadfully. In addition, there were the mounting hospital bills. Apparently, there was Canadian legislation during the polio epidemics that assisted families that had a polio member, but it didn't apply to those from the Yukon. As a result, Gary's parents were faced with a bill of $2500 a month—impossible for a family of limited means. It was the Royal Canadian Legion that became their advocate with the University Hospital, urging the powers that be to settle for 50 cents on the dollar. The hospital was reluctant, but finally acquiesced. Once the McPherson family had lived in Alberta for a year, hospital expenses were then covered by the province.

Getting an education was not that easy either, but thanks to the Correspondence School Branch and the help of volunteers, Gary made it through Grade 10. He liked reading, but couldn't turn the pages himself. As a young teen Gary and his roommates ventured further and further afield, building up a wide range of interests, including amateur radio, which opened up the outside world to him. He became a Ham Radio operator and this hobby eventually lead to his involvement in Wheelchair Sports. He and a few of his roommates started their own computer software company called Pro-Data Services Ltd. in the University of Alberta Hospital. The Company eventually grew in size, forcing a move into an office downtown. At one time in its ten-year history, Pro-Data employed twenty-seven people.

Through yet another friend, he and his roommates became interested in horse racing. So much so, that the enjoyment was continued even in the hospital where he and his friends, affectionately called "the boys", collectively designed a horse racing board game called Pounding Hooves.

His future began to take another direction after he read and followed up an ad in *The Edmonton Journal* for Junior Chamber of Commerce Week. Gary joined the organization and through the Jaycees he took several courses in self-development and personal growth. These courses included public speaking, parliamentary procedure, and leadership training. In 1971 he was elected to the Executive of the Edmonton Jaycees and soon became Secretary Treasurer. Said Gary, "I gained confidence because people accepted me for what I could do, not for what I appeared to be—disabled." Access to Jaycee meetings was difficult at best, and eventually it became one of the factors in his decision to leave the Jaycees, which he did regrettably.

Gary learned to travel and loved it. In 1967 he and a good friend went to England to visit Gary's grandmother, and in 1972 he and his brother Scott (now deceased) went as observers to the Paralympics in Heidelberg, Germany. These experiences subsequently became a catalyst for Project Hawaii, a trip that took a good part of the University Hospital's polio ward to Honolulu—about thirty people in total, thirteen of whom were either ventilator- or oxygen-dependent. This took meticulous planning. Gary is quick to commend Wardair and its employees for their caring attitude and attention. It was Wardair's corporate example that eventually allowed this unique trip to become a reality for many people that had not experienced travel since getting polio.

Friends were always important to Gary, and they often played a big role in helping him to become involved in various activities. He has been described by a very close friend as being "like a magnet", because he is viewed as being wise, courageous, and enterprising.

Gary now has an extensive background in the voluntary sector, having spent more than twenty years in wheelchair sports administration. For eight years he served as President of the Canadian Wheelchair Sports Association (CWSA). He has been recognized for his work with numerous awards and has been inducted as a member of both the Edmonton and Alberta Sports Halls of Fame. On November 16, 1995 the University of Alberta Senate recognized his contribution to the community by awarding him an honourary degree of Doctor of Laws.

In June of 1998 he officially joined the University of Alberta where he became the Executive Director of the Canadian Centre for Social Entrepreneur-ship in the School of Business. In addition, Dr. McPherson is an adjunct professor in the Faculty of Physical Education and Recreation.

Now perhaps you understand why this book would be incomplete without including Gary's story. He's written a book titled, *With Every Breath I Take*, about health and self-responsibility that is based on his personal experience with the medical system. In addition, several articles and books have been written about him.

Once They Get to Know Me,
They See Past My Handicap

SANDRA KEMP-PATERSON

MY LIFE CHANGED DRASTICALLY on a hot sunny day in August 1959 at the age of twenty-one months. I was playing in our backyard when stung by a bee. I developed a fever and my legs swelled. My mother called the doctor who, in those days made house calls. He diagnosed these symptoms as polio, and explained that the symptoms had nothing to do with the bee stings. They rushed me to the Montreal Children's Hospital where they did a spinal tap. This confirmed that I had polio. I was then taken by ambulance to the Alexandra Pavilion. They strapped me to a board to keep me straight because I was paralyzed from head to toe, only able to move my eyes back and forth. They would only let my parents hold me for short periods of time.

Memories of those days come in flashes. I remember lying in bed moving my hands, and all of a sudden there were doctors and nurses all around me. That must have been the moment my hands and arms started to recover. I also had extensive surgery on my legs and was in a body cast for about four months. When the cast was removed, the doctor found little pieces of cardboard that I had shoved between the cast and my body to relieve a terrible itchiness. And my legs, having been straight for so long, were really sore when they were bent. My mother would give me special baths to help my skin come back to normal. I remember having physio at home after the cast came off.

There was a feeling of guilt in my family because I hadn't been vaccinated. Like now, there were some people who were fearful of the vaccine. I have friends who won't have their children vaccinated and I look at them and urge them to think again. But you can be assured—my daughter has been vaccinated.

I spent a lot of time in Ward 5K at the Children's, and the person who made a big difference in my time there was a volunteer named Paul Lindsay. I'd really like to see him again. He took pictures of everybody and had them posted on the walls in the hallway of 5K. He spent a lot of time with us. I remember one day there was a blood drive in the playroom on 5K and I wanted to go. The nurses tried to convince me that I wouldn't like all the needles and things. So

Paul distracted me completely by doing a photo shoot.

My legs are paralyzed, especially from the knees down. I also have a curvature of the spine. This scoliosis must go back to when I was a child because when I came out of the hospital, I had a back brace for two months. Then when I got the leg braces, I stopped using the back brace. I guess I couldn't use them both. When I was twelve, I had surgery on my spine. A few days after the surgery they put me in a wheelchair and told me I should get some fresh air on the eighth floor roof garden. All I wanted to do was lie down. For this procedure they had made an incision on my side, removed a rib, collapsed my lung and passed very close to the main artery. This procedure (Dwyer) was done by a doctor from New York. Apparently the operation was taped. That was in 1972 or 1973. I have never seen this tape but hope to do so someday.

My mother used to do certain movements with me at home—I guess you'd call it physio. Two or three days a week I would have physio at school. My sister and I were very close even though she was older than me. She spent a lot of time coming to the hospital to visit me because my mother had other children at home to care for. I overheard her whispering to a friend, "Don't treat her differently—it's just her legs." I remember zooming around the house on my hands and knees; my mother had a hard time getting me to wear my braces. She must have asked my brace maker to tell me how important it was to wear them because the next time I went to Slawner's I was duly lectured. But even at school I would get in a wheelchair whenever I could get away with it. It was easier to get around.

I went to the Mackay Centre for Deaf & Crippled Children known to us as the School for Crippled Children, for the first nine years of my education. I felt sort of like the odd man out, because not many people there had polio. I felt lucky to be one of the more able students. Those, like myself, who got around on crutches were known as "walkers", whereas most of the other students had cerebral palsy or muscular dystrophy and got around by wheelchair. I was in Grade 2 at the Cedar Avenue school the year they moved to what is now the Mackay Centre on Decarie. Mr. Grey was my bus driver. I remember there was only one elevator at the Cedar Avenue school which carried two wheelchairs at a time. We had to take turns to get up into the school. The new building on Decarie is very accessible.

When I had completed Grade 9 it was recommended I attend a regular school. I was the only one at my new high school who was handicapped. I was very fortunate however, that one of the girl's brothers had been to Mackay with me and she was my saving grace. She knew me, which gave me a sort of "in". I remember one day at school two boys were fighting in the hall. One of them was pushed into me and I fell. A girl came running and picked me up.

She started scolding the boys, and they were so apologetic. To help avoid falling I would walk alongside walls and push against the wall to slow the possible impact. Both my knees are straight and I never quite know in what position or where I'm going to land.

A few months after I started working I remember a colleague had asked me if I wanted to play tennis after work, which proves that once people get to know me, they see past my handicap, and even forget.

I have recently been diagnosed with post-polio syndrome and no longer walk with my braces and crutches but use a manual wheelchair to get around. Quite possibly I will have to use an electric wheelchair to minimize the stress on my weakened arms that have begun giving me so much pain. Since my childhood I was able to get around and do almost anything. Polio was something that had occurred in my past and I got on with my life. Now some forty-odd years later, I have begun feeling new pain and weakness. As a result, some changes had to be made: I now work part-time and have learned how to pace myself so that I don't get too tired.

I am married to a fantastic man, Andrew, who has had to put up with a lot more than other husbands do because of my disabilities. I am also the proud mother of a very bright and talented fifteen-year-old daughter, Rebecca.

My biggest frustration with polio was being unable to walk with my baby in my arms, especially being unable to soothe her when she had colic. I had to teach my husband how to hold our daughter properly, how to pat and comfort her. Not being able to do these things myself really hurt. "If only I could do it." The first three months of being a mother were the most difficult for me. Rebecca often says she wishes she had a brother or sister. I'm quick to respond, remembering those early years, and say, "I'm allergic to babies."

Polio has made me strong and given me a pretty good perspective on life. I look at people differently and try to understand what they are feeling and what obstacles they have had to overcome.

My Experience of Polio

VICTOR-LÉVY BEAULIEU

MONTREAL NORTH. Pie-IX Boulevard. I'm getting off Bus 139. A weird soreness rips through my ribs. I'm having terrible problems breathing and I'm barely walking, afflicted by a persistent pain in my back.

I see a drug store; I enter and ask for Aspirins. A man in white hands them to me and I continue on, seeing lights jumping before me. I return home, Castille Road, and I don't even have the energy to take off my clothes. I stretch out on the sofa, my head feeling heavy, like a block of steel. I feel as if I'm slowly drowning at the bottom of a well.

It's a horrible feeling.

I close my eyes and fall asleep.

When I wake up, it's morning. I have a very bad headache, and I feel sick. I throw up a few times and am forced to stay in bed. I'm unable to eat, I have a fever and I'm barely aware of what is happening around me. My mother calls for the doctor, who examines me.

"I don't know what I can do", he said. "I could easily be wrong, but from the symptoms, I am led to believe that it is an attack of poliomyelitis ... weakness in all the muscles, fever, headache, pain in the neck, vomiting".

"Should we send him to the hospital?" asks my mother, who is suddenly anxious.

"No, I don't think so. I would advise you to do nothing, to wait. One never knows. In any case, let me know if he gets worse".

All day I had nightmares: blue whales would spurt viscous liquid onto my face; walls of stones would pour over me; gigantic slices of bread with huge velvety paws would make me sick. I couldn't eat a thing. My stomach wouldn't cope and my mother seemed desperate.

It's now evening and my temperature has gone way up. The doctor comes back quickly and advises me to have a complete medical exam in the Maisonneuve Hospital. As I had never been in a hospital before, I am anxious and afraid.

My brother André's old Plymouth races through red lights and pouring rain and gets me to the hospital in less than fifteen minutes.

A nurse leads me to a door, at the end of a hallway: Emergency. In spite of myself, I begin to tremble. I'm really scared. What are they going to do to me? What is becoming of me? In my excited state, a myriad of thoughts, each one more improbable than the next, jostle my mind, causing me to panic.

They lay me out on a stretcher which is so high I spend the night worrying about falling off.

Doctors and nurses work around me, examining every part of me and taking blood samples. While an intern questions me as if I'm a criminal, another nurse approaches me with a strange apparatus that makes me shiver.

"I'm going to take your blood pressure".

She winds a sort of air-chamber around my arm, waits a few seconds, then whispers a few words I can't understand into the ear of the doctor. He turns back, looks at me, then says to the nurse: "I hope you are wrong. I'll check".

The nurse was right. The doctor leaves suddenly, for what reason, I can't guess. He returns shortly with a few colleagues who begin one at a time to examine me. One shrugs his shoulders, another scratches his chin. They seem perplexed. Hammer taps on my knees, on my ankles and elbows, questions, answers, doubts, uncertainty, more blood is taken.

I ask for a glass of water and swallow two pills of heaven knows what.

Everything I see is a jumble and even my sleep is full of nightmares that make me break out in a sweat.

Another morning dawns. A specialist comes to examine me. He prescribes a lumbar puncture. It is a procedure that requires taking a few drops of spinal fluid. The pain is atrocious when the needle enters. Perhaps I screamed. I can't remember.

A little later in the forenoon, a nurse comes to advise me that I would be transferred to the Louis Pasteur Hospital, a medical institution that specializes in poliomyelitis.

I am thunderstruck.

It's two in the afternoon when I arrive at the Pasteur on Sherbrooke Street. There is a thunderous wind. I feel more dead than alive with my stomach in turmoil. Once again, they examine me from head to toe. I shall always remember the doctor who had a scar under his chin.

On a stretcher, dressed in a gown that was provided by the hospital, they take me to Room 322 where I have to wait fifteen minutes before getting into bed. They had forgotten to warn the personnel of my arrival. There was no bed, no mattress, no sheets. I waited in the corridor by the door, in despair of ever being able to go into my room.

Finally they put me on a mattress with a plank underneath, no pillow, with feet supported against a wood panel. The plank under the mattress prevents muscle collapse and scoliosis (lateral spinal deviation). As for the wood panels at the foot of the bed, they were to protect the feet, the tendons and ligaments, against possible weakening. Sandbags and a thin cylinder of material placed under my knees assure flexibility and impedes undesirable positions which would result in a withering or deformation of muscles.

Stretched out on this bizarre bed, I admit, I look wretched.

I begrudged being ill at a time in my life when I needed all my strength. I feared losing a scholastic year and missing my sister's wedding. Nonetheless, I remained optimistic, not fully aware what polio was and to what degree I was affected.

The poliovirus is strange in that it is one of the most known and at the same time unknown of viruses. It's best known because of its physical characteristics, its prevalence, and its resistance to antibiotics. What isn't known (or wasn't at the time this was written) is how the virus is transmitted. Poliomyelitis, a disease of summer months, is an illness felt by muscles that experience deterioration. Important to note is that it is not an illness whose symptoms are similar from one person to another and whose outcome is predictable. Each case is unique and requires specialized care.

It has now been ten days since I was hospitalized. The danger period is over, but I can't get used to the hospital. I'm in a daily routine of overwhelming loneliness. Severed from my normal life with healthy people, I am frightfully aware of my weakness and my powerlessness. In effect, I can do nothing for myself; my existence is entirely in the hands of nurses and doctors.

How different life can become all of a sudden.

I ask myself questions even though I know that they are useless, ridiculous. "Why me? Is this illness going to make me handicapped for the rest of my days?" I ignore it still, but they tell me that polio often leaves its victims considerably damaged. I am truly frightened and the answers I get from the nurses are not reassuring.

However, I am aware that my moaning and tears will change nothing, that I have polio, and that my only option is to try to get better. I tell myself that it will be a lengthy cure: interminable weeks, maybe months. But I am ready for any sacrifice to regain my liberty, my family, and my friends.

Each morning a nurse subjects me to what I call the martyrdom of Sister Kenny hot packs, a treatment consisting of wrapping the affected limb in hot wet compresses. The heat accelerates circulation around the muscles, calms and lessens the pain in the weakened limb. It seems that it is the most effective and simplest procedure for recovering muscle mobility—indispensable for recovery. The results of this treatment, for my case, are astonishing.

Slowly I regain my strength. I'm aware that I am a shadow of what I was, that I tire over nothing, that I don't eat or eat very little, that I am easily irritated and extremely nervous. But there is progress nonetheless.

The doctors bluntly refuse to let me walk. I am not even able to sit in my bed in order to avoid spinal deformity. I am reminded that certain polio victims are permanently paralyzed because they did not listen to the advice of their doctor. No doubt this is an exaggeration, but I can honestly write that most of the advice was at least partially true. One doesn't play around with polio.

Shortly after my arrival at Pasteur, near the end of August, at the height of the epidemic, two young boys joined me, Nelson and Roch. Luckily for them, their polio had been detected in time. But Nelson wouldn't stop crying which kept us awake all night. He had terrible pain in his legs that no medicine was able to help. Exhausted by his suffering, he slept all day.

A few days later I was transferred to the 4th floor, Room 411. I was overjoyed. I'm going to be able to leave in a few weeks. My inactivity is coming to an end!

But I am quickly disillusioned.

I find myself in a room with an old man, dressed all in white; I am troubled to see he is missing a leg. There's another young man in his twenties who, sitting on the edge of his bed, appears so hostile that I cry. Hidden by my covers, I want to die.

After two long days we still haven't talked, each clinging to his place. Then, all of a sudden, for no reason, we started talking to each other.

A nun, the first I've seen in the hospital, enters our room and asks me what I would like to eat for breakfast. I ask about the menu.

"Cereal and cornflakes", she answers very seriously.

We burst out laughing and we watch her leave profoundly vexed.

And it is then that the old man suddenly shows his extraordinary volubility. He started telling us all he knew about the hospital—the food, the personnel, medications, physiotherapists, patients and the nuns.

"Here," he said, "you eat turkey and you have the indigestion of a calf!"

I personally have a good reason not to like the meals because I was not allowed to sit up and had to eat lying on my back, with the help of straws. Being a lefty by nature, it was practically impossible because of the paralysis of my left arm to eat properly, to write, or to kill time.

Boredom leads to my asking for school books so that I could study sciences, math and Latin.

Bernard and Normand, my two roommates, go to physiotherapy. They leave me alone for hours. Fortunately an aide comes to visit me often enough and encourages me as best she can. She tells me anecdotes that help me forget for a while the inactivity that is so wearing.

I've now been in the Pasteur for a month. My sister got married while I was in the Hospital; I spent my birthday on September 2 in utter silence. My friends came to visit me, but I felt their discomfort.

As for me, I still am not allowed to get up and walk. The doctor says that in my case rest is preferable to physical exercises. I am condemned to this idleness and it frightens me. I would like to run and to dance. I am still not fully aware of what has happened to me.

My left arm, withered, won't move. The deltoid muscle no longer functions; my biceps are lifeless; the trapezium, the infraspinatus and supraspinatus muscles are also considerably weakened with the result that any muscular effort on my part is out of the question.

As soon as I start trying to use my arm, it hurts. Every day a physiotherapist has me doing exercises in bed; she is trying to prevent further contraction of my muscles. I'm as rusty as an old iron bar; my muscles no longer respond to my will.

I ask the physiotherapist a lot of questions. Being German, she understands little of what I am asking, so I am none the wiser. But I have come to understand that I am in this for the long haul before recovery if indeed I ever recover.

That afternoon they come to get me on a stretcher. I am taken to the swimming pool for certain exercises. Hot water (100°F) makes movements easier because the body doesn't have to cope with gravity in the water. But I am only taken there three times; there are patients in greater need of water therapy than me.

Slowly I recover my physical shape. But my arm, to all intents and purposes, fails to move.

I fully understand the gravity of polio when I see for the first time an immense iron contraption in the hall. It's an artificial lung, known as an iron lung. Patients are enclosed in it, except for their heads, to assist their breathing. They say the iron lung is a last resort. One can't look at it without shuddering.

In the room next to me there's a woman who has been dependent upon an iron lung for three years. Another woman, young and five months pregnant when she was admitted, is to give birth in October. She also lives in an iron lung. I fear for her; I fear for the child to be born.

We are ten young men and women whose ages vary from sixteen to twenty-two years. With the exception of Marie-Paule who has Guillain-Barré Syndrome (an illness resembling polio but different because there is no muscular atrophy), we are all polio patients. We all became friends. In the evenings we visit each other, play cards, talk. Lucio is from Sorel, Lise and Bernard from

Montreal, Marcelle from St. Alexis de Montcalm, Réal from Sherbrooke, Lucien from Trois-Pistoles. Conversations were interesting, varied, and sincere.

But gradually we understand that this cannot continue. We are friends without a tomorrow. Lucio will leave first and leave us his wonderful drawings; Bernard will leave us soon for the Rehabilitation Centre; Lise will return to her family.

We are happy to know they will soon be released but we nonetheless dread the thought of their leaving us. But how we would like to be in their shoes, hurriedly pack our suitcases, never again to see these soulless walls, these airless rooms, all these unfortunates who have no hope!

But then again, we can do nothing because we rely upon the men and women in white.

I'm becoming discouraged as the second month in hospital goes slowly by. Despite all the exercises I've been doing, the weights I lift, in spite of the extensors that I pull, my arm refuses to move appreciably. My movements are awkward. I still don't understand the upheaval that polio has bestowed upon me.

Saturday morning. The doctor comes into my room and warns me that I shall have to wear a special apparatus on my arm if I don't progress in the coming two weeks.

I am despondent. I can't even study.

The two weeks pass and my muscles strengthen. The doctor advises me to become an outpatient of the Institut de Réhabilitation on Darlington. I am so excited that I accept right away. At least I can now be with my family. I would at last have my freedom.

I leave the Pasteur Hospital one Saturday morning, seventy-one days after being admitted. As of the following Monday, I am admitted as an outpatient to the Institut de Réhabilitation.

It has now been six months that I have gone to the Rehab at three in the afternoon for my physio treatments, which last an hour and a half.

Will I fully recover?

I don't know. I must wait another three months to be certain. Poliomyelitis is a capricious disease. Healing cannot be taken for granted. One must work, and work continually. I know all about that.

In all probability, I shall not be able to use my arm fully before next autumn. As for my studies, I am going to pursue them in the evening and in that way will not completely lose my school year.

All in all, I am lucky to have pulled through this episode with polio so unscathed, even though a couple of injections of the Salk vaccine could have spared me the experience.

Quebec author and playwright Victor-Lévy Beaulieu is founder of the Festival de Théâtre de Par Chez Nous and the publishing house VLB.

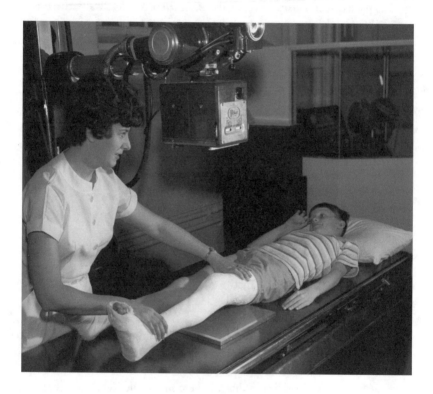

Plaster casts, sometimes covering most of the body, were a painful reality for many polio patients.

Despite Polio's Limitations, I Functioned Normally

PÈRE YVES GAUDREAULT

I THINK I HAD POLIO twice in my life. The first time, I was very small but old enough to remember. My mother always said that I had polio back then, but I really don't remember much, just a few details. I was about three or four years old. I was living in La Malbaie, Quebec, where I was born. I was the second in a family of seven children who had not all yet been born when I had my first occurrence. Since we were all about a year apart, there were at least five of us when I got sick. Something that I remember particularly well was that my parents put a small bed in their room and I slept with them, on that small cast-iron bed. I think the polio was fairly severe. Once I tried to raise myself on my legs but they would not support me at all.

I don't think I was hospitalized during that time, undoubtedly because La Malbaie was located some ninety miles from Quebec City and we did not have a hospital in our town. So I stayed at home and our family doctor treated me with some sort of serum.

I have always doubted that this was a polio serum. I put most of the episodes with the serum out of my memory. It seemed more a folktale than the truth, as I have never heard of its use except for the treatments prescribed by my doctor. My skepticism about this infamous serum dissipated, however, when many years later, I read the book *Polio's Legacy*, where it was mentioned that in the 1920s a serum was indeed used in cases of acute polio. Apparently the serum was a concoction of monkey blood and human blood. The human blood came from individuals recently cured of polio. The serum was given by injection. Of course later it was determined that the serum was not at all effective, but at least it caused no harm. Knowing that I received the serum injections then, in all likelihood, I had polio when I was a tot. To the best of my knowledge, I did not develop any lasting effects from this first encounter. But I have never been a "Tarzan" and I remained rather thin. I do not think that had anything to do with the polio.

The second time the poliovirus struck me was more memorable. In 1964, when I was thirty-five years old, I was living in Tanzania, Africa. I was a missionary priest with the White Fathers of Africa, living in a small city very close to Tabora in the heart of the country. I was assigned to a large seminary, a kind of faculty or school of theology for Africans. I arrived in October 1961.

It was during January 1964 that I started to feel very sick and feverish. I thought that I had the flu. I was wrong. Accustomed to playing tennis every weekend, I said to myself, "I'll play tennis despite the flu. This will give me a good sweat and break the fever." I played a set with much sorrow and misery and finished only because my opponent was very competitive and wanted to win. I remember very well that when I returned to my room, I walked with great difficulty and felt sore all over. I lay down, feeling terribly sick.

The next day I was taken to a small hospital in Tabora, which was six miles from the seminary. A young English doctor with very little experience saw me. This hospital was really badly equipped; let us say it was more of a dispensary than a hospital. But at least there was a doctor, which was wonderful! I was put in a bed and some blood tests were taken. During the night I felt a very strong pain in my right leg and I could not sleep until in the early hours of the morning when the pain finally subsided. I think I was able to sleep a few hours.

I woke to the alarm clock, and while getting up, I fell. My right leg did not function any more. It was really very weak and it could not support me. I had no idea what was causing all this trouble. The doctor continued with his investigations while focusing on the paralysis in my right leg, which he suspected was polio. He called for a lumbar puncture and that confirmed his suspicions. Poliomyelitis.

It was out of the question to return me immediately to the seminary because, in all likelihood, I was a carrier and contagious. On the other hand, he didn't know what to do with me. At this time in Africa the majority of people with polio did not go to the hospital. They remained in the bush and became crippled or died. If they did survive and were paralyzed they would get around by pulling themselves on the ground. So, even though polio was in the bush, the doctors did not see many cases, and this doctor didn't know what to do with me.

There was this one time when the young doctor came to me with his medical books in hand, and said, "You are not progressing according to the data in my books."

My condition worsened, albeit gradually. In the beginning I thought that only my leg would be affected, but the paralysis moved into my upper body. I was in a lot of pain and my strength was fading. Finding a comfortable position was impossible. Obviously, I did not have an adapted bed in that small hospital, so I had to use pillows to try to find some comfortable positions. I asked for sleeping pills at night, but even if I did sleep, even a little, the pain was so strong I could not sleep soundly.

One night I called for help several times but nobody came to my bedside. After a few hours, an African nurse finally arrived.

He told me, "We heard a leopard."

The corridors of the hospital formed an external veranda and there was the bush all around. Wild animals could enter and make their way around on the veranda. So when the staff heard a strange noise, they would not dare move for fear of being attacked.

There was not only the threat from wild animals but also from an unstable army. During my hospital stay there was a rebellion by the Tanzanian army. There were two battles, one in Dar es Salaam, the capital, the other in Tabora. As this was only three years after independence, there were still British senior officers in the army, and the Tanzanians had had enough of being controlled by the British. They decided to put the British on a plane and dispatch them. As this gesture was not acceptable to the government, the army responded to the government with a rebellion. The President disappeared.

There was a news blackout for three days and there was no way of knowing what had happened or what was going on. We later found out that the army had taken control of Dar es Salaam and Tabora and anarchy prevailed.

Before long, the army showed up at the hospital. The soldiers circulated with their rifles. They looked nervous. Paralyzed and confined to my hospital bed, I was periodically informed of the developments.

Suddenly one day some friendly people burst into my room and shouted to me, "You must leave! It is too dangerous! We don't know what they are going to do to the whites!" I wanted my rescuers to return me to my seminary where I lived with blacks, which I thought would have been much safer than putting me in with other whites. They replied that this could not be done because there were roadblocks everywhere.

They took me in their arms, I was in pajamas, and whisked me out to a waiting Jeep. As we left, I watched a soldier approach with a weapon in hand. He looked very nervous. I do not know if he was doped up or not, but he never drew his weapon on us, and we drove away.

The decision instead was to find me a place in some remote house. This plan was not so much for my safety, but more for the fact that I was contagious and could not be placed where there might be children. There was this old English army major who had taken his retirement in the bush. They decided to take me to his place and I could stay on his sofa. I had no medication or treatments for the pain.

The Major was very nice to me. He spent a lot of time telling me stories of his experiences and other things about the past. It wasn't easy for me though. I could not always listen, as I was feeling terrible and could not find a comfortable position on his sofa. The pain would not go away. But, despite my discomfort, the Major remained quite attentive to me.

The pain persisted until the last day on the Major's sofa. It was in the evening when an African priest, a Tanzanian from my community, took the Major's Volkswagen and brought me back to the seminary where I had a room on the ground floor, but still no doctor or medication available for two full days.

Finally, the Head of State, Julius Nyerere, asked for help for the country from the British who had troops stationed in nearby Kenya. British planes made some low passes over the cities to frighten the soldiers and when the planes landed, the soldiers fled.

The way was clear, and I was able to return to the hospital where I stayed for another three weeks. Things were looking up. I met a young doctor with a child in his arms, proof that the doctor thought that I was no longer contagious. He told me that I could return to Canada. My trip was prepared and I was to leave, confined to a stretcher, in a DC3, first to Uganda.

I could not walk at all. I was completely dependent. I could not even raise my arms and I had trouble sitting. In Uganda, an ambulance took me to the hospital for a layover. The following day, I set out again, still on a stretcher, to Amsterdam. There I went through the same scenario. An ambulance took me to a hospital where I stayed for a night. The next day I was taken, as always, in the ambulance to the airport. But this time, on the way, a car struck the ambulance, and the shock was so violent that I lost my pillows.

We arrived at the airport only to discover there would be a slight delay. The attendants decided to put me on the plane anyway. The problem was with an engine that had some sort of breakdown and had to be repaired. That also meant that the plane would not be heated. We were in the middle of February! An employee gave me some small covers, the thin ones distributed to passengers on aircraft. The repairs took more than an hour to finish while I froze in the cabin. I was so cold that when the plane finally took off I felt that my toes had frozen.

People came to speak with me during the flight. They were very sympathetic. Then, I had to go to the toilet. I requested some help from a steward. He supported me while I braced myself on the backs of the seats on the way to the rear of the plane. I got there, but I couldn't get back. All my strength was sapped, and it didn't help that I was too tall to make my way through the low interior of the plane and I couldn't support my hunched over body. Finally the stewards had to carry me in their arms.

I arrived in Montreal where an ambulance was waiting to take me to the Hôpital Pasteur. I was placed in the ward for infectious diseases where I remained until the following June.

My mother always worried about me. She came to see me after my arrival at the Hôpital Pasteur. She knew that I always wanted to be a missionary, and when I was young and dreaming of my future work, she would often say to me, "You will come back sick." With that I would jokingly tease her by assuming the bent over posture of a lame missionary. When she did arrive, I took up that old joke, and bent myself over, and said, "We always knew that I would come home like this."

Everyone treated me very well at the Hôpital Pasteur. At first I was put on bed-rest which made sense since I had been through a lot. I was exhausted from the plane trip halfway around the world, the leopard, the army coup, and the old English major.

When treatment started, I was encouraged to do the Sister Kenny treatments—light exercises in my bed followed by rest and hot packs. Occasionally I was taken for a hot bath.

When I was able to leave my room, one of my first exercises was to crawl on all fours over the mattresses in physiotherapy. This became a bit of a game, as there were many children in the treatment room while I was crawling around. They made the experience unforgettable. We turned the crawling exercise into a kind of dog-eat-dog game. They bit at me, we barked, they jumped on my back. They called me "Mon Oncle". It was wonderful.

One of my brothers brought me a television set. At this time it was not like anything that we have today, but it was television. The children would get together in my room when Michel Louvain was on. He was a popular singer, but I had no idea who this Louvain was. He certainly was well known to the kids, and after a few months of watching Michel Louvain, I could say that I knew him very well too!

Some of these children seemed not to have fathers. With all the time that I spent in the hospital with the children, I suppose that I became a sort of father figure to them. Sometimes, when I needed to go in my wheelchair for my exercises, certain kids insisted that they sit on my knees for the trip to physiotherapy.

I graduated to the parallel bars, and it wasn't long before I was able to manage on crutches. The following June, my brother-in-law took me home to La Malbaie. My mother was still rather young at this time, and my brother had a beautiful country cottage on the edge of a lake, so Mother and I spent a splendid summer from June to September by the lake.

Sometimes I rolled myself down to the lake to bathe because I still could not walk without crutches. My right leg and my back were too weak. I said my mass sitting, after which I felt exhausted. However, I never gave up on my exercises that I followed with a determined passion. I exercised outside on the grass when the weather was good or inside the cottage when it was bad. It didn't matter where. All that mattered was that I exercised. Slowly I regained my strength.

At the beginning of my experience with polio, I wondered whether I was going to die. When I realized that I wasn't, I found myself watching the paralysis progress, and I wondered how far it would go. I was very fortunate that I did not have bulbar poliomyelitis because there was no help in the African bush for people suffocating from the paralysis of bulbar polio. There was no question of using an iron lung. There weren't any. Almost certainly I would have died.

When I think back on my days in Africa, I can see that I was content to live in the present. I focused on adjustment and did not think about what was coming, about what could happen, or whether or not I would recover from my paralysis. I lived in the present and that helped me. The people around me also helped. Everyone encouraged me. That filled me with confidence. Confident or not, after doing my exercises, I was always too exhausted to worry about the future. I could not even wonder whether my life as a missionary was over. Admittedly, I always kept hoping that I would start contributing again.

Certain people sometimes told me, in a rather pious way, "The good Lord loves you because He has sent you this test." This kind of piety infuriated me. I would answer, "This is not my kind of belief. God does not amuse himself by sending this business upon us. I believe that God has been with me in my suffering and has helped me to stay here, to do all that I can for myself, and to get myself back to health. He is not amused."

Anyway, I returned to La Malbaie and was growing stronger by the day. By September I was moving under my own power. My reliance on my crutches was waning. In January I was strong enough to join the Novitiate for the White Fathers in Chomedey, Laval. I wasn't perfect by any stretch of the imagination. While there all I could do was focus on continuing my exercises. I broke my routine a couple of times a week when I would go to the Dominicans for hot baths. But other than that, it was exercise.

At the Novitiate from January through September I made no intellectual efforts. I read very little. Certainly I had many opportunities for discussions and for meeting with people, but I never had the strength for concentration on talk or banter. My physical exercises were exhausting. I just had no power for talk. Without energy, I just let myself be carried by events. For me, I had to concentrate exclusively on exercise and nothing else mattered.

By September the desire to start reading returned. At first I found reading difficult. The concentration wasn't there and it took an eternity to finish a book, but I felt that now was the time for mental exercise. I read more and more and took in some lectures while continuing my physical regimen.

Finally I managed to walk without crutches!

With that I took up, little by little, some of the activities of my professional work. When my superiors judged that I was sufficiently healthy they asked me to take a position on the Faculty of Theology in Ottawa. It was July 1965, one and a half years after my second episode with polio.

Work filled the day. I rested after dinner. In the evening, I reserved some time for myself to exercise and swim. Joy of joys, I was feeling well enough to start playing tennis again. I did not have my old coordination back, but I did feel rather powerful. I could run a little. There was a slight problem if I bent my leg a little too much. I would often fall. This wasn't all bad because, I must admit, I could turn this weakness to my advantage as a psychological tactic to destabilize my opponent.

I stayed in Ottawa for six years, where I had the opportunity to talk a lot with young people, and especially to listen to them. This experience led me, or encouraged me, to take a master's degree in social psychology in Chicago.

Later, I was named to the General Council of the Society of White Fathers in Rome. I spent six years in Rome, during which time I traveled just about everywhere in Africa, Europe, and even Australia. I practically forgot that I had had polio. I certainly had a little less endurance than the average person, but I did not regard myself as an invalid or handicapped.

By 1981, I was back in Tanzania. I lived in the bush and as there was some time for leisure, I started to garden with the students. I worked often and as you can imagine I spent a lot of time hunched over my garden. One day in 1983 I tried raising myself when I felt a very sharp pain in my back. I was about a mile from the house but it might as well have been ten thousand. I was in excruciating pain. The car ride back home was unbearable. When I did drive up to the house I nearly crashed as I could not raise my legs, and the pain was so intense that stopping the car was near to impossible. I could barely work the brakes. I remained immobilized by pain in bed for several days.

Since then my back has been fragile. I have had to pay special attention to it because those pains return with little provocation. An inadvertent twist and I am hobbled.

In 1984 I transferred to Kenya. I was able to play tennis but little by little my performance worsened. I was less coordinated. I started losing! And the pounding on the hard court surface woke the agony in my back and legs.

I had to slow down.

By this time I had come across some articles about post-polio syndrome, and I started to consider that it could be part of my problem. It was time for a rest. I thought that I would return to Canada for a vacation.

In 1990 I packed my racket in my bag which was promptly lost on the way home. I decided that then was as good as any to give up my career as a globetrotting tennis player. It was for the best. In Canada I felt that certain muscles weren't responding the way they used to respond, and I was falling more often.

After my Canadian vacation, I returned to Tanzania. In 1993, the Society asked me to go to Uganda. It was at this time I noticed that I was having a little more difficulty climbing stairs. My right leg was becoming weaker. I felt more tired. I needed to rest more often. Sigh … I had to accept my new limitations. I felt obliged to refuse.

Three years later, my superiors offered to send me to Jerusalem to oversee the house there. I would have liked to go, but there were so many stairs in that house and the streets of Jerusalem were so uneven that it was just impossible for me to go there. Instead I came back home to Canada in 1995.

What was the positive side of this disease? I think that it brought a larger capacity for self-ridicule and for not taking myself too seriously. I remember when I was thirty-six years old doing physio, and like a dog on a mattress exercising with a dozen handicapped children playfully nipping at me.

I have been very fortunate despite the fact that polio struck twice in my life. I have avoided serious negative effects and have managed to do all that I have done. Polio did not leave me seriously handicapped, although it did decrease some of my strength. There was a time when my colleagues didn't want to entrust certain responsibilities to me because they were apprehensive about my physical limitations.

As of this writing, my symptoms have escalated to weakness in my right leg and general fatigue. Walking on uneven ground, with or without my corset and orthopedic support on my right leg, causes a lot of trouble for my back. Taking a leisurely stroll in the woods, for me, is no different than walking on a sandy beach; they are equally difficult. I manage with the strength and ability that remains, while living a comparatively active life.

Every now and then an astute observer may remark that I walk with a small limp. Good. As strange as it may seem, one difficulty that I have relates to the fact that my physical problems are not always apparent. Often I find that I need to explain why and when I cannot do such and such a movement. It is not easy for many people to comprehend that I cannot remain seated for long, or remain standing long for that matter. At mass, for instance, I can celebrate a mass supported by my corset and leg brace, but two masses are out of the question.

There is no doubt that my strength continues to wane. Aging is taking its toll too. Looking back over the years, I must admit I was adversely affected by polio. I had physical limits, But despite all of this I functioned normally and I have contributed to society in a way my vocation called me to contribute. I couldn't ask for anything more. The Lord has been with me in my difficulties and I have been able to lead a full life and continue to do so. I have enjoyed being part of Polio Quebec since 1995 when I attended its conference in Montreal, and took on its presidency in 2000 for two years.

A Cheerful Heart Is Good Medicine

MARIO DI CARLO

IN RIBERA, a minuscule town in Southern Sicily, another young toddler, just beginning to take his first steps, became a victim of the poliovirus at the age of thirteen months. He was never to walk again on his own. It seems odd for most North Americans who had already been receiving the polio vaccine for years, to hear about a polio infection occurring in 1963. Nevertheless, the illness left the young boy, yours truly, with severe generalized paralysis. Everyone felt totally helpless. Not even our "Sicilian friends" with all their "ammunition" could do anything but watch and pray.

In the fall of 1964, my parents, my new baby sister, and I immigrated to Montreal. My parents thought they could receive better help for me in Canada while improving the overall family living prospects. Their focus was on the family. Their strict and demanding approach was balanced with unmistakable expressions of encouragement, challenge, and affection. Although they couldn't prevent the dreaded disease from knocking at our door and settling in, they did all they could to give me the best second chance available, including Canada, a land of opportunity and ingenuity.

I began my treatments at Ste. Justine Hospital for Children. For years I couldn't walk and did not use assistive devices. I remember simply dragging myself on the floor or walking on all fours. I developed calluses on my fingers from the amount of time I spent on the floor. When we went out, my parents would either carry me or use a baby carriage. How can I forget the embarrassment I felt using a carriage at the age of four or five? "I'm not a baby!" I thought. As physiotherapy began, my parents were helping by following up with my exercises at home. Unfortunately, the language barrier with the medical team made it difficult, at times, for them to fully carry out the physio appropriately.

By the time I was six, I had recovered sufficient strength to begin using full leg braces and heavy metal Canadian crutches. I hated that. They were extremely bulky, intrusive, and uncomfortable. I often preferred just being on the floor without them. I felt freer! Moreover, as often occurs with polio victims, I had developed, through the years, severe scoliosis. This forced me to also wear a rigid surgical corset. With this weighty "armour" on, I'm sure I was bullet-proof! I looked like Robocop.

Fortunately, time has its way to help people adapt to new circumstances. As I began to wear my armour, I developed an appreciation for my newly found independence. It wasn't perfect but it beat being carried or using a baby carriage. At home I would try to do away with my annoying braces and corset and just use the crutches. Indeed, I had developed sufficient strength on my left leg and arms to be able to roam around with my crutches only. I was still using the rest of my apparatus most of the time, but by then I had become very skilled with my crutches and we became inseparable.

Before long, it was time to go to school. Although apprehensive, I was ready for the challenge. My parents found a school adapted for and dedicated to handicapped children. Everyone had a visible or invisible physical challenge. This experience taught me a new reality: I became aware that I wasn't unique in my circumstance and that there's always someone in a worse situation than me. I also realized that some invisible ailments can be worse than the visible ones. Yes, I saw many of my schoolmates and friends pass away in my childhood with cystic fibrosis, heart disease, brain tumours. At the end, I felt viscerally fortunate that, contrary to my friends, I was dealing with a visible monster and I became determined to fight it "till death do us part". And so began a journey of introspection, education, and the pursuit of challenges.

I completed my schooling and graduated with a Bachelor's degree in Fine Arts. While still in university, I married the exceptional girl I had met two years prior. I was studying and working part-time while she had a full-time job. Within a few years of our marriage, we were blessed with three wonderful children. I soon completed my studies and began my career.

The positions I have held since graduation have typically been in customer service and sales. From my second year of working full-time, I quickly went up the ladder, gradually holding more and more important leadership positions in various corporations. I went from supervising twenty-five people to directing hundreds of people with multi-million dollar budget responsibilities. I began traveling extensively, going from meeting to meeting, working long hours and bringing work home, all while juggling family responsibilities. In addition, I got involved in serving on various boards and in our church community. I was determined to push my limits!

All this was exhilarating. I thought my balancing act was pretty good; I thought the monster had vanished, until my body warned me otherwise. A few years ago, signs of deterioration began to emerge. Pain, weakness, and fatigue gradually became omnipresent. I could not ignore my setback. I was losing control. The fight or flight response system kicked in and I had to react. Do I ignore the warning signs and keep going or do I gather ammunition and confront the symptoms?

In my experience with the church and spirituality, I learned some invaluable lessons. For instance, the Bible declares "There is a time for everything, and a season for every activity under heaven" (Ecclesiastes 3:1). Later in that same chapter it is written "What does the worker gain from his toil?" and there is "A time to keep and a time to let go." These thoughts spoke to me. I had to put aside my natural (or acquired) instinct to want to push forward. I realized my lifestyle was hurting me. I had to let some things go. I stopped some of my extracurricular activities. That wasn't enough, the symptoms were still there.

Recognizing the inefficacy of my actions, I actively sought medical attention. A series of tests and treatments was prescribed. Eventually, the treatment included the use of a scooter, installation of an elevator in the home, and a more radical change in lifestyle: I stopped working. That was probably one of the most challenging times of my life. It was quite a sudden deceleration for a car going full speed. At the time of this writing, I have been on a leave of absence for a year, during which I have received many treatments and a surgical intervention. An ancient proverb affirms "a cheerful heart makes good medicine" and so I try to take a daily dose or two of this concoction.

I am indebted to my family and friends for their patience, affection, and support. I feel honoured and privileged to have served in various capacities thus far. I haven't thrown in the towel yet and do not intend to do so. I am encouraged by the words of an old prophet: "The Lord will guide you always; He will satisfy your needs in a sun-scorched land and will strengthen your frame. You will be like a well-watered garden, like a spring whose waters never fail" (Isaiah 58:11).

Polio Quebec Association thanks Mario for being president of the Association during the challenging year of readjustment caused by the symptoms of his post-polio syndrome.

We Can Succeed Only if Surrounded by People Who Believe in Us

KIM

I WAS BORN IN CAMBODIA in 1971. When I was but four months old there was an epidemic of polio in my country. I had not been vaccinated, since the vaccine was administered only at age six months.

Obviously, I do not remember the beginning of the disease, but my mother has told me that I had a severe fever and she had to take me to several doctors before finding out that it was polio that was making me sick. One of those doctors gave me some sort of an injection to lower the fever, after which I could not move any more. I did not cry any more. I did not drink. I was like a vegetable. My mother did not understand anything. No one knew if the paralysis had been caused by the injection for the fever, but we were led to believe that it should never have been given.

Medicine in Cambodia was not anything like in Canada. The doctors were not as well qualified. Still sick, I was returned home without any treatment. I did get some treatment, however, when my mother took me to a Chinese doctor who gave me several drugs. He also inserted needles in my legs until I cried. Gradually, strength returned to my arms but not to my legs.

In Cambodia there was war and it was necessary to flee the country. I had an uncle who lived in France and he invited us to go there. My father had been killed in the war so it was just my mother and me who immigrated to France when I was ten years old. When we arrived, I was taken over by Immigration and they transported me to a hospital to see if there was something there that they could do for me. I underwent two surgical operations, one for my legs and one for my left arm. I wore plaster casts for two months, during which time I stayed hospitalized flat on my back, unable to sit up. My knees, which had become frozen in a bent position, were now surgically straightened and I was able to be fitted with braces and crutches, and finally able to walk short distances.

At any rate, I was in France and I did not speak a word of French. This was a major problem, but at ten years old, one learns quickly. During my hospitalization people were very sympathetic to me and I have very good memories. The nurses and the doctors helped me a lot and we became friends. Everything went very well for me despite having to adapt to a new culture, which required much effort.

Because of the war in Cambodia, I was never given an education. Cambodian children did not go to school during the war. I actually began my schooling after my arrival in Europe. In France, handicapped children did not go to a regular school, and as I was in need of rehabilitation, they put me in a rehabilitation centre in Alsace, close to the German border. It was there that I began both my rehabilitation and my schooling. I was still ten years old. I concentrated very hard on learning French.

We can only succeed if we are surrounded by people who believe in us and by those who are willing to give us a helping hand. Me? I was surrounded by therapists, physiotherapists, doctors and even professors, all of whom supported me. They respected my pace and rhythm in life. For the first two or three years I found it very difficult to be away from my family. I had to learn how to walk with braces, to learn a new language and to adapt to different food practices, especially to eat cheese, an unknown in Cambodia. I had to learn to eat like a European. Our financial means were very limited and it was the French government who assumed all the medical bills and expenses.

I stayed in France until I turned twenty-two. By then one of my aunts was living in Canada and my mother wanted to be close to her family. We arrived in Quebec in 1993, and I had to make yet more adjustments. I knew nobody, having left all my friends in France. I still mourn. I had to do something to continue with my university studies.

To be in one country one day and another the next, this change obviously would not be easy for anybody. I could never thank enough the people who helped me, not just my family, but many of the people I met, especially those among the handicapped. If one does not receive a little push, a helping hand, then one cannot follow in rhythm with society. I must admit that at university there were times that were very difficult for me, mostly in connection with adapted transport. Just moving from one place to another was hard. When I began my courses I was a little disappointed with the University of Quebec at Montreal. The integration services for the handicapped were not in place. I found myself, for example, with two courses on the same day in two different buildings, one on Ste. Catherine Street and the other on Berri. How was I to get around? To overcome this problem I did not take more than one course per day, but I had to go to school four or five times a week. Integration services have improved since I started, and there have been big changes as a result of the complaints from handicapped students.

During my childhood, before I was ten years old, I did not feel different from the other children since in Cambodia everyone was in the same situation. We were all at war, handicapped or not. In France, however, it was different. During my stay in France, I lived in a sheltered environment. It was not until I left for college that I had my first contacts with non-handicapped people. And I did have difficulties coping at a regular school. I felt out of place. I did not know how to approach others and did not know how other people were going to react to me. I suppose all handicapped people are a little afraid of that. The 'glance' does not disturb me any more because I am accustomed to it. I think that there are people who cannot look at a handicapped person, yet there are others with a strong sympathetic disposition. These are situations with which one must learn to cope. After all, one cannot change everybody. No one ever said anything that really wounded me. But people were nevertheless hurtful because, in fact, when people avoided me, that in itself was hurtful.

I use a wheelchair in everyday life, even when I am at home. When I went to university, I would wear my braces so that I could get from the wheelchair to the toilet. My right arm has remained paralysed. Since I cannot use my right hand, I use my left hand for the majority of activities. As I have been handicapped since the first months of my life, my mother has the tendency to be over-protective of me. She is always afraid for me when I plan to go somewhere and she insists that I tell her what is going on which I do to keep her from worrying.

I am naturally very reserved. It is not because of polio that I do not have a very active social life. Each one has her own personality. I like to go out, but I choose my friends carefully. I would say that I am a rather solitary person. Perhaps this is due to the fact that I am an only daughter. As for my quality of life, I do not think that there are any problems there. I would like to go out more often, but I am restricted by adapted transport. I have friends who get me around. When I think of all the people dying of hunger in the world, I consider that I have nothing to complain about.

I have a few years before I finish my studies. I am quite aware that there will be problems with regards to employment. Access will be a primary constraint to employment. There will doubtless be architectural barriers. I will not be able to work just anywhere. In addition, some employers might not be ready, I imagine, to employ a handicapped person in their firm.

Would that people start thinking more about the needs of the handicapped, and I don't mean thinking only about those with polio. Each time I go out I have to be sure that the place I'm going to will be accessible to wheelchairs. When I lived in Paris, buildings were not accessible, and I'm sure this resulted in the institutionalization of the majority of handicapped people.

This also puts a strain on the families of handicapped people because it forces the family to assume the burden of mobility. The French do not have the same social structures like the ones we have here. When I arrived to Montreal, I was a little astonished to see that there were handicapped people walking on Ste. Catherine Street. In Europe, one rarely sees that. There, when handicapped people went out, they would go in defined groups.

I think that it has been my destiny to be wheelchair-bound. It has taught me always to persevere although I do still come across times that are difficult. Sure, there are certain people who are ready to help. When in class, for example, several people don't even have to be asked. But helpful people are not always there.

If I had my legs, undoubtedly, my life would be different. I would travel more. You wouldn't find me spending all my time studying in the university library. I would do many things if I could move more. I would surely do everything that everyone else is doing. I would be entirely free to come and go as I pleased and I would not have to depend on adapted transport.

Since this interview, Kim has graduated and is fully employed. She drives a car that accommodates her wheelchair. She is also the auditor for Polio Quebec.

I Got Polio for One Good Reason

KARMA BURKHAR
as told to Sally Aitken

KARMA'S FAMILY was living in Southern India. That is where she got polio, in a village four hours by bus from the train station, with a further forty-eight hours by train to Delhi, where treatment might be available. Karma and her father Sonam came to Canada by means of a ministerial permit to get treatment for her polio. They were the subject of a CBC Newswatch documentary in 1994 when Karma and her father were threatened with deportation because their visas had expired. The documentary shows Karma's teacher, Ida Ripley, and her Grade Three classmates at Bancroft School, who were among the hundreds of people who wrote letters of support. A lawyer volunteered his help, and thanks to the efforts, good will, and common sense of various people, Karma and her father are still in Montreal, and have been joined by her mother, brother, and sisters. After collaborating on this text, Karma completed her CEGEP years at Dawson College and is now a full-time student at McGill University.

A day after my third polio vaccination, I got a fever and my legs crumpled when I went to the bathroom. I kept getting worse, so I was taken to the hospital. At first they didn't know what was wrong with me. They consoled my family by telling them not to worry. Everything was going to be okay. But eventually they realized that it might be polio. There were about ten others in the community who had similar symptoms. What else could it be? That was in 1984, in Kollega, Southern India. I was two years old.

My mother says that I was like a little baby. I had to be propped up on pillows. My hands were clutched together, with my fingernails digging into my palms. My whole body was paralyzed, my left side being more affected than my right. My father asserts that my upper body got better because my grandfather, who is a shaman, performed some Buddhist rituals over me. My grandfather became very ill all of a sudden, and wasn't able to continue his rituals. My family believes this accounts for the paralysis in my hips and legs. To get around I would put my feet on the floor, with my legs fully bent, clutch my feet with my hands and move my feet forward! I never crawled. To get places, my mother would carry me on her back. My parents took me around to different places looking for cures. Despite assurances that something could be done, nobody was able to help. I don't remember much about those times, except that my friends included me in their games and treated me normally. Because of polio I became close to people, especially my grandparents. I guess I was sort of spoiled. My Uncle Ngodrup (who was an interpreter for the Tibetan government) wanted me to come to Canada for treatment, and he found it possible through Judith Cutler in Montreal. She was an active member of the Rijpe Dorjee Centre. In 1986 we ran into Stephanie Colvey, another Montrealer who was on assignment in India at the time. My father, my uncle, and I were on top of a bus going to visit my grandparents in Mirik in Northern India. It started to pour with rain, so I was lifted through the window of the bus and found myself on Stephanie's lap. Stephanie was an old friend of my Uncle Ngodrup. So for a growing number of reasons, Montreal was chosen as the place for me to go with my father to get some help with my polio. It was also the home of the wonderful Shriners Hospital. It took over two years to get sponsorship, ministerial permits, and financing organized.

When my father and I came to Montreal in 1989, I went straight to the Shriners Hospital. My first doctor, the Chief Surgeon, believed I would be able to walk. I was presented to a diverse group of specialists, all of whom believed that walking was out of the question. But through the insistence of my first doctor, I was given the opportunity of having physiotherapy treatment with Joanne Gibbis. With the help of two long-leg braces attached at the waist, and a walker, she got me walking. It was a lot of work for both of us. I've since had two rounds of surgery. The first was a hip-releasing procedure achieved by cutting some tendons in my groin. Now I'm much straighter.

A few years later I had surgery on my back because of a painful 81 percent curvature in my lower spine and 51 percent at the top. The operation was in April 1997 at the Montreal Children's Hospital. Dr. Arlet said, "Wow! I like it." The surgery cured all my old pain. This was such a relief, but not for long. My former pains on the lower left side came back and caused me to twist around in my bed, never able to get comfortable. This was corrected by the surgery only to be replaced by a generalized pain in my lower back and arms. It feels like someone is pressing my back and arms, even when I am lying down. The surgeon hoped the pain would go away, but it didn't. Dr. Cashman thinks it might be fibromyalgia. Most of the medical team didn't expect I would be able to walk following the back surgery. It's true that I now use a wheelchair almost all of the time. But my balance is good and I can walk if I have to, even though it's very difficult and I'm scared of falling. I'm told I shouldn't do too much and at the same time I shouldn't do too little.

I began my life very happy. I had a great childhood. I do not remember much of it, but I do remember being happy. After Grade 6, I began to change a great deal. I became very angry at the world because I realized for the first time that whatever I had to do, I had to fight for it. It is one of the saddest things that a person can ever learn. It was during this same period that I realized how people truly viewed me. I became aware after I accidentally ran over a teacher's foot with my wheelchair. Instead of just accepting my apology, she began to humiliate me in front of the whole class. It was around the same time that I realized that was not the first time I had heard such words of seeming hatred and ignorance. That incident helped me remember my Grade 4 teacher who told me that I should be in an institution instead of attending a public school.

High school was a complete nightmare for me. Though I remember good moments in elementary school, I cannot remember anything good about high school. It was a time when I learned some harsh lessons in life. I divide my teachers into two groups: those that just saw my disability and those that went out of their way to make my life difficult because they decided that I must have an easy life because of my disability. Most of my teachers thought that I used the elevator as an excuse for being late for class. Once when I arrived for lunch early the vice-principal sarcastically pointed out that I could make it to lunch on time but not to class. Though I did not reply, I wanted to ask the vice-principal how many times he saw me arrive early for lunch.

Unlike so many people, I have the ability not only to accept but at the same time to conquer. After having overcome many obstacles, I know that I can do whatever I want. There are so many people in my generation who are busily trying to fit in. These people do not have ideas of their own nor do they have passions. Having a disability means having a different outlook on life. It is no longer black and white. Meanwhile, I am very fortunate. Society does not have any expectations of me, and most importantly, society does not expect me to conform to fit their ideals. Thus, I have the luxury to become my own person. And I think that is the greatest gift a disability can ever give a person. I think my polio has had an extremely positive effect on my family. I believe I became handicapped for one good reason, and that was to change our family's Karma, causing them to come to Canada to a better life. If they had stayed in India, opportunities would be very limited.

My handicap is sort of like my Karma, which after all is my name and means "good or evil action". It is a means of making a difference for my family. Some people believe that I am handicapped because I did something bad in my past life. I am handicapped to benefit the lives of my family members, to give them an opportunity that they would not have had were I not disabled.

My disability has made me a more patient and understanding person.

Being in this situation, I am more aware of the abuses that are going on around the world. I feel passionate about people's rights and the environment. I do not believe in sitting aside while human and environmental rights are being abused. My disability has made me more reflective and carefree. I do not seek the approval of society before I do what I please. A lot of people think that I wish I could walk, but that is definitely not true. I'm used to being in a wheelchair. It has become an important part of who I am. And I'm able to achieve much more than people can imagine.

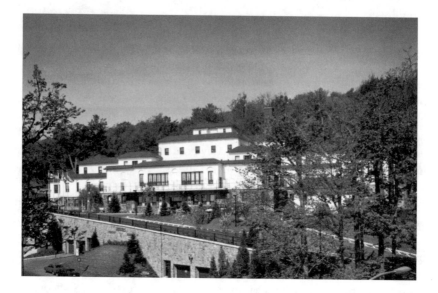

The Shriners Hospital on the slopes of Mount Royal, Montreal.

Three

Polio as Experienced by Family, Friends, and Community

The following accounts recognize the impact polio had on the supposedly unaffected members of the family and the community. Parents pitched in to the limit of their ability to help their child recover, siblings were often jealous of the attention being given the brother or sister who had been stricken with polio, and husbands or wives were faced with a totally unexpected role as caregivers. Not all marriages bore the strain. Children, however, seemed to be totally accepting of parents with a polio handicap. They would defend their mother or father's physical difference if challenged, as if they were blind to the physical difference and accepting it in their range of normalcy. My son for instance learned to walk with his limping Mum as a model, so he limped too. Once I recovered from the surprise, I explained, and he understood that it would be better to walk like his father.

Across Canada in 2001 there were outpourings of gratitude for the mothers who fifty years earlier had started going out on the hustings to canvass for the March of Dimes. They became known as the Marching Mothers. One of them recalls a year in Hamilton when people were encouraged to put their coins on a chalk line in the centre of Main Street. Five miles of pennies and dimes were collected this way. But in subsequent years they reverted to going door-to-door because it was less risky. The need to collect for the March of Dimes and Easter Seals continues. Their help for young and old includes people affected not only by polio, but many other handicaps.

Michel Robitaille

A Well-adjusted Life

[by Sally Aitken]

In 2001 the anniversary of the Marching Mothers was celebrated in various ways across Canada. In Regina, Saskatchewan, a beautiful commemorative garden outside the Legislature Building was dedicated to them. British Columbia proclaimed March as the provincial Post-Polio Awareness Month, and in Ottawa mothers were awarded a medallion of an enlarged commemorative dime for their years of volunteering. The design was adapted from a photograph provided by the March of Dimes.[1] A registry was also launched in an attempt to record all mothers and fathers who have "marched" over the years collecting millions not only for research but also for all types of helping devices for people with a diversity of handicaps.

Then there were the countless mothers and fathers whose lives were turned upside down when faced with caring for a handicapped child. For the most part, it was done with love, perseverance, and determination to challenge their handicapped offspring to their maximum recovery.

An excellent example was Marcelle Terreault, the mother of Michel Robitaille. Michel died in 2001, and his wife Pierrette DeGuise volunteered to share with me the meticulous record of Michel's history with polio compiled by his mother Marcelle. She also had a collection of clippings and pictures related to polio and her son Michel's involvement as a chosen polio person in the 1940s and 1950s. These were used for news and March of Dimes/Easter Seal campaigns. Marcelle was by her son's side from the beginning of his polio episode on September 19, 1943 at the age of four, and cared for his well-being throughout her life. Judging from her diary of Michel's medical episodes, her duty as a mother rarely let up. It would seem that her son had every contagious disease there was, as well as a long episode with jaundice. Then there were twelve operations to correct problems caused by polio. She encouraged home learning[2] so that her son would keep up with his age group scholastically. He did more than keep up. He excelled, with marks in the high 80s.

His career was varied. He wrote wonderful songs, started a rock and roll orchestra, and even performed in Carnegie Hall in New York. He took a mechanical design course, was a credit manager, and finally, the proprietor of a video film studio. He married three times, had three children, and spent seven of his latter years in a motorized home with his wife Pierrette happily avoiding winter and moving to different warm-weather campsites every two weeks. Summers were spent in Compton, Quebec. When he realized his strength was giving out, he and Pierrette sold the motor home and moved into a Montreal apartment. Needless to say, Marcelle can't be credited for all these successes, but she gave Michel a supportive and loving launch into a well-adjusted life.

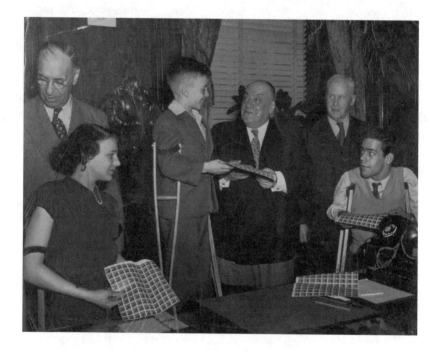

In this 1949 picture, Montreal Mayor Camillien Houde is buying a sheet of Easter Seals from eight-year-old Michel Robitaille.
Richard Arless Associates.

James Valin

Maybe My Dad Didn't Go to War, but He Fought in One of the Great Battles of this Century

[by Stewart Valin]

My father was born Sydney Franklin. His name didn't stay Sydney Franklin; he changed it to James Valin. His mother was Suzie Franklin; his birth certificate said it was Miss Franklin. I usually don't believe everything that I read. It could easily have been something else. After all, Dad was born out of wedlock and it was during religious times. This wasn't exactly the best situation to be born into. He was born of a sin and it was wise not to be too enthusiastic about advertising one's religious shame. So that is why I am not certain about her name, and I really don't want to know it. His father was unknown—the paperwork was certain about that—so there was no shame for Mister Unknown. Nonetheless, Dad was born January 12th, 1917.

Dad died eighteen years ago. He was sixty-two years old. He told my brother Glenn that each year he lived was a bonus. He said that considering everything, he should have died when he was three years old. Quadriplegic, and spending time in the iron lung, his hopes for life were slim back then. He had been orphaned and he was dying. Had it not been for his guardian angel, Mumzi Levesque, who during his greatest need adopted him, polio surely would have claimed the child who was to become my Dad. As much as his life represented courage and strength extraordinaire, it was Mumzi Levesque's legacy of love and firm resolve that brought the battered, wounded boy to life.

I met Mumzi only once, not long before she died. Dad brought me and my brothers and sister to meet a true angel. Details are long lost, but the blur of a woman sitting in front of a yellow window, proud, and trying her hardest to look her best, remain. There was not much more than a bed, a table and the chair she sat on. The room was down a long corridor. The floors were dark wood. Nuns nursed her now, the Grey Nuns I think. Her days were coming to an end.

I suppose Dad wanted to show off to Mumzi. Alive, married with children, he wanted to show her the fruits of her labours. It was a great gift for her. His story, I suppose, is also her story. She was the rare tiller, working the earth for broken bodies and a dying soul. She nurtured my Dad's life where polio sought otherwise.

An early picture of Dad dressed in Indian costume gave a hint of his polio. Standing in heavy shoes, there is a soft outline of leg braces holding him up under his long pants. Unless I was to have known he had them, I don't think I would have noticed. He looked normal. But there was something wrong with the little boy's body. His hands. They were weird. They reached out from under the long sleeves, a little longer than seemed normal, and they turned a bit, showing the backs. The fingers curled. He was paralyzed. He was proud and happy to have his picture taken in his brown Indian costume.

Mumzi worked Dad very hard. Exercise and more exercise eventually brought the legs back and the braces were gone. Part of my Dad's legend has the braces hanging somewhere on the walls of St. Joseph's Oratory with the canes and braces of other thankful souls. His arm muscles never really caught on. They forever hung from his shoulders. Not lifeless—they could be used a little—but they kept that telling flatness and twist.

To me, Dad was different. I didn't see his funny ways of doing things as different from other dads. It was style. Actually, it wasn't until I was about nine years old that I noticed anything unusual. My friends Jeff and Steve and I were playing while Dad mowed the lawn. They stopped and stared at my Dad. He had no shirt on. It was hot. Other fathers were without shirts doing work also. Our next-door neighbour was out without his shirt. His back showed off scars from shrapnel wounds from combat in World War II. There were deep gouges in the muscle under his scars. They were big and frightening. It must have hurt.

"What's wrong with your Dad?" they asked.

"Nothing."

They stared. "The bones are sticking out of his shoulders."

I looked, then said, "There's nothing wrong. He's always like that."

"There's no muscle. He pushes the lawn mower with his stomach. What's wrong with him?"

"Nothing." I was devastated.

Other fathers were using their arms. Driving the mowers forward with giant muscles. My Dad pushed forward on his legs. His scrawny arms hooked to the handles. They braced the mower between his stomach and chest. At the end of each thrust he trudged back dragging the mower with nothing arms. The momentum of the mower brought the handles to his chest again. It hit him with a grunt. The blades whirled then he thrust forward again. He couldn't push-pull a mower like other fathers. Watching him seemed like an eternity.

Dad was different.

"He had polio."

"What's that?'

"I dunno. It made his arms like that."

"He should wear a shirt."

I stared. He should wear a shirt. Those shoulders weren't like giant scars from war wounds. Bone sticking out, no chest, no muscle: without scars or war stories these are things that make folks stare.

"Oh, he had polio."

It's not like, "Oh, he got shelled in a tank."

No, he didn't.

It takes me back to even earlier times. When I was seven years old, in the big field beside St. Monica's Church in Montreal my Dad trooped my bothers and me onto the grass. Here we learned to play football. Hut hut hut, and we would be running down the field and Dad would fire off a long spiral pass. He grunted. He grunted when he threw long before professionals grunted. It helped propel the ball down field. He cheated. As with the mower, he couldn't use his arms much. He hung onto the ball, pushed forward on his legs and twisted. He grunted. His arm swinging, he'd release the ball and off it went. A forward lateral, the best forward lateral you'd ever see, but not allowed.

"Dad. That's not allowed."

"It's the only way I know how."

He had his own way of doing ordinary things. It was normal in our house never to talk about polio. It was there—at the dinner table, the morning shave, brushing hair. Who had to talk about it? We were experiencing it. I'd watch without saying anything. To brush his hair, he had to swing his left arm across his stomach—it was big—and catch his right elbow. Holding the elbow in place, and bending it, he would lower his head to meet the comb. With long strokes of the wrist he groomed his black hair. He always had a full head of hair. With bright blue piercing eyes, he was a handsome man who took good care of his appearance.

At the dinner table getting the salt and pepper was—different. One day I imitated him and it's the only time I remember him getting angry about his way of doing things. I thought it was neat, the way he moved his arm across the table to get the shaker. It was like "letting your fingers do the walking through the Yellow Pages." He would walk his hand on two fingers across a stretch of table to the salt. Grab hold and then pull back. So I did a walk on the table, past my plate, around the butter, over to the pepper. Well, that didn't go over too big.

"What da hell are you doing?" he boomed.

"Getting the pepper."

"What are you doing?"

"I dunno. I was getting the pepper."

"Never do that again."

"Do what?"

"It's not how you get the pepper," my mother shouted.

"Dad does it that way."

"You don't. Your father does it that way because he has to. You don't."

"You've got goddam good arms. Use them!"

Part of growing up male, I suppose, means imitating Dad, if you're fortunate enough to have one. At the time, I didn't think imitating my father was wrong. It felt right. But I can imagine my rather large family, six kids, going out to a crowded restaurant. Squeezed together at tables pushed into a line, heavy into chat and fight, and getting the butter or something by walking our hands on fingers. Sixteen hands scrambling around the table, a busy ant colony collecting food and carrying it back to home plate. I see what a spectacle we would have made. So I don't imitate my Dad at restaurants, but every now and then at home I take a little nostalgic walk around the table—to get the salt.

"What are you doing Dad?"

"I'm getting the salt."

"Why are you doing that walking with your fingers?"

"My Dad did it this way."

"Why? It looks stupid."

"He had to. He had polio in his arms and he couldn't reach for the salt. So he walked."

"Really." And off Julia's hand went on a walk.

"It's weird," she said.

"We never do it in restaurants."

I was in church, attending mass. At the end of mass, the priest, who knew me, came to me and told me to go straight home. My Dad had had a stroke.

In the emergency room, the doctors and nurses stared at me with a bit of fear, sorrow, and anxiety. Passing through the doors I noticed him in the first bed.

"Oh, God."

He saw me and shouted, "Stewart."

Dad had facial ataxia pretty bad. His head was fairly still but his eyes bulged and rolled around. He couldn't control his tongue—it was swollen, sticking out, and licking his lips furiously.

"Oh, God." I looked back at the emergency room staff. They shook their heads. "We're transferring him to the Neuro."

"Dad." I stroked his hair. "You've had a stroke."

Hearing what was wrong, the ataxia suddenly stopped. His face was peaceful. He stared.

"Feeling any pain?"

"I've got a bad headache. It really hurts."

"How're your legs?"

"They're okay."

They weren't moving. I looked at the staff. They shook their heads. They didn't know the extent of the paralysis. It was too early to tell. Maybe they wouldn't be paralyzed at all. His arms were working—sort of. He stared at me. Dad made it to the Neuro but there he had another bleed. In a coma, he died in two days on February 26. Mom said he had told her he wouldn't want to be paralyzed again. He'd rather be dead. "He couldn't do it again," she said.

Mercifully, I suppose, he died.

Maybe my Dad didn't go to war, but he fought in one of the great battles of this century. Poliomyelitis never drew a battle line between grown men; it fought a cowardly war against children. Hospitals, homes, and orphanages—this monster stalked its targets and struck without mercy. My Dad, carrying deep wounds from polio shrapnel, won no medals, but was one of the great heroes of battle.

Neil Compton: A Tale of Love and Courage

MARILYNN VANDERSTAY

IN THE SUMMER OF 1955, on his thirty-fifth birthday, Neil Compton, chair of the English Department at Sir George Williams University, fell victim to polio. After six months in an iron lung, Neil was able to go home. Recuperation was long. A year later after struggling in a small apartment, Neil and his wife and three young children (Chris, Vanessa, and Sarah) were able to move into a Westmount home with the help of some generous friends. It was a home with a formidable wooden wheelchair ramp built to access the front door.

The floor in the back room was reinforced to hold the rocking bed that Neil slept on, as well as a heavy oxygen tank. The rocking bed performed automatically, providing the same enabling pressure that would be exerted by artificial respiration. The always-innovative Neil, however, learned to breathe without a respirator using the unique glossopharyngeal breathing technique (commonly called frog-breathing). While awake, Neil was now free of a respirator and was able to return to his position at Sir George. Neil had learned about frog-breathing from an American magazine. A physio helped him learn the technique and make it work, although it was new to her and had not been covered in her training. A fellow polio patient and subsequent lifetime friend had the same breathing problem but did not learn this frog-breathing technique and consequently was never able to return to work.

In 1960 his wife left him and their three children, and Neil lived in fear of having to put the children into foster care. A serendipitous visit from the twenty-three-year-old daughter of a family friend changed everything. Gabriel McCulloch was passing through Montreal en route home to England after teaching in the United States for a year. Although she had no experience with cooking, she agreed to stay on to manage the household.

A year later she added a position teaching classics at Sir George Williams University to her responsibilities. Neil and Gabriel married in 1962 and over the next few years the Comptons became a larger family with the arrival of two daughters. Having sex in a household with three teenagers whose visits to the kitchen were unpredictable at any time of day, as well as coping with the dynamics of Neil's rocking bed, which had to be turned off, was transformed into formidable acts of love for Gabriel in particular. Neil admitted to his devoted wife, "you make me feel like a human being." Their first-born is appropriately named Victoria! And then there was Miranda.

For Gabriel and Neil those ten years were eventful. Every year they would throw open the French sliding doors in the living room/dining room to host parties for the entire English department. Guests would number up to seventy-five in an evening. Later Neil and Gabriel would discuss the parties while Neil rocked in his bed off the kitchen and Gabriel cleaned up. A peak moment for Professor Compton was in 1967 when he presented an honorary Sir George Williams University degree to Dr. Gustave Gingras of the Institut de Réadaptation de Montreal. Dr. Gingras had played an important role in Neil's adapting to his polio limitations.

Although he used an ordinary wheelchair at home, while at the university he used an electric chair that had been imported from England. It offered two speeds forward, and one back, and was operated by a joystick which he controlled with his one functioning hand, his left, although even that functioned to a very limited extent. He had to be helped physically to cough, and have that arm in a sling to blow his nose or eat. He slowly and painfully learned to write with a curious device invented to replace the ability of his fingers. The University arranged a scholarship for a student who in return was a personal assistant to Professor Compton, enabling him to manage his personal and teaching tasks while away from home. Most of these assistants remained friends with Neil and his family; two actually became their daughters' godparents. What a bonus this helping position was to the scholarship. It gave to both parties more than money could buy.

In 1971 Neil had an accident in his wheelchair caused by a malfunctioning elevator in the Hall Building of the University. On the day of his accident he was making his way to the Faculty Lounge on the seventh floor of the Hall Building. His assistant asked if he wished to be accompanied, but he declined. It was to have been an easy ride, what with his electric chair and an elevator. But no. The elevator stopped about three inches above level ground. Unaware, Neil confidently put his chair into reverse. He tipped backwards and cracked his skull. Although the visible wound was minute, the massive brain hemorrhage required a thirteen-hour operation at the Montreal Neurological Institute, and it was doubtful he would survive. Dr. Bertrand was his surgeon, and of memorable help and support was resident Dr. Stephen Nutik. Gabriel was immensely impressed by the whole Neuro team.

Neil was at the Neuro for about six months and recovered as best he could, but he was left with severe brain damage. Homecoming encouraged recovery, but it was limited and he realized he wasn't going to be able to go back to work. His daughter Sarah was a pillar of support to the family at this time.

Neil's final months were marked by frequent and sometimes harrowing emergency visits to the hospital for cardiac arrest and a tracheotomy. It was a challenge to get the hospitals to understand his special needs arising from polio. He was exhausted. He gave up and died at home in his sleep, ostensibly from incipient pneumonia. That was in 1972.

The unshakeable Gabriel carried on and when her daughters were of school age she sent them to the arts school that was then called FACES. (It is now known as FACE.)

In another serendipitous meeting over a problem one of her daughters was having at the school, Gabriel met co-founder and principal Phillip Baugniet. In 1977 the two were married and soon increased the family by two more children, Rebecca and Joe. Around that time Gabriel Baugniet was featured in an article in the Montreal *Star*; "The Greying of Motherhood" was about mothers having babies after forty.

The Baugniet family, with four children remaining at home, continued to live in the house with the ramp, housing various grandparents through the years. The house remains the same as it did forty-five years ago, except the sliding doors no longer slide. Neil's extensive library is shelved as it was. The couple continues to host an annual party. Grandchildren play where their parents once did. Only the ramp, which was finally taken down in 1982, has disappeared.

This essay was inspired by an article written for the Westmount Historical Association.

Gordon Armstrong

This Was All New to Me and Very Frightening

[by Iva Armstrong]

It's time the heroes of the polio era were brought to light and their story told. This is how I experienced polio living with one of its survivors, my husband Gordon, and I'm only too glad to have the opportunity to share my story.

In July 1947 Gordon and I were visiting the Swails in Grenville. Gordon didn't feel at all well. He had a severe pain in the back of his head. That night he didn't sleep, so the next morning we returned home. He insisted upon driving. Once back in Shawville, we went to the doctor who counseled us to go home, that Gordon was probably suffering from the flu. Gordon went right to bed, but the next morning he couldn't move, so we phoned a young doctor, Dr. Bruce Horner, who had recently taken up practice in Shawville. He came to the house and it wasn't long before he was carrying my husband to the car. He took him to the community hospital in Shawville. From then on life was difficult.

Gordon was twenty-seven at the time. I was twenty-four. We had been married for three years and had a little girl called Joan. When Gordon went to the hospital, Joan could speak one word—"car". By the time we came home, she was talking. We really missed that part of her life.

Before going to a Montreal hospital, Gordon spent time in the contagious disease hospital in Ottawa. Unknown to me then, they didn't expect him to live. An iron lung awaited him in Ottawa. Luckily he didn't have to use it. But when the time came to leave, the question was, where to go? Being paralyzed from the neck down, it was clear he needed intensive physiotherapy. So we traveled to Montreal in a train's baggage car. Gordon was on a stretcher. An old school friend, a nurse, accompanied us. Being met at the station in Montreal by a Royal Victoria Hospital ambulance was an unforgettable moment. This was all new to me and very frightening. Even though I had my little suitcase in hand, I had no idea where I was going to stay. Fortunately a cousin from Verdun welcomed me and I slept on her old chesterfield for two or three weeks. And then a friend of Gordon's who taught school in the Shawville area took me in. She was living then in Montreal North. From two in the afternoon until eight at night I was at the hospital, working whenever possible with the physio-therapist. I recall how terrified I was when I had to go home after dark on those autumn nights up St. Laurent Blvd. on the creaky old streetcar and having to walk quite a distance.

At the Royal Victoria Hospital Gordon was first admitted to the main building and then moved to the Montreal Neurological Institute and Hospital across the road. Dr. Wilder Penfield and a whole crew of doctors visited him. Heaven knows what they were looking for. They used the Sister Kenny treatment of hot packs. I helped the nurses apply them. And this treatment continued when Gordon came home. We had a large copper pot on the stove. Gordon's mother and I would take the towels out and wrap his limbs in them. The heat and the moisture helped, I guess. We also persevered with the physio because the nurses had taught me what to do, but, oh my, those legs were heavy.

Thanks to our good parents and sisters, our daughter Joan was very well looked after during our time away. I came home once to see my daughter and when I returned to Montreal, found that Gordon had developed pneumonia. His breathing remained weak and he never regained the ability to cough.

When we returned to the farm, he could do little but lie on the bed. When it was time to try walking, his dad would get on one side, his mother on the other, with me in the rear. One leg was always a little bit better than the other, and I was the one that would move the weak one forward. We did this routine for a long time and his strength improved a little. One of his friends brought him a wheelchair and that was his first chance to sit up. It took years before he could do anything without help, though. My parents had a place in town, so we moved in with them from the farm where we had been with his parents. I was then able to return to my teaching.

Gordon learned to walk, but with great difficulty. He could just barely make it across a room. His right hand was mercifully strong. Once he could manage to get into a car, he was able to drive. He was very disciplined about doing the exercises that had been prescribed so that he would recover as much strength as possible. This didn't leave him time for much else. At the end of that year I began feeling sore, first of all in my thumb, then my foot, and hip. I went to my girl friend's home for a week of rest and relaxation. I was young and strong then. All my aches and pains disappeared and I've never looked back. I give Gordon a lot of credit. He was an easy patient. He never got out of sorts.

Gordon's working life outside the home ended when he got polio. His first job was in the Calumet mines, but he left when he bought himself a good-sized truck. We used it only once (to help my sister move) before he got polio.

The truck had to be sold. Given the geography of rural life, I don't know if he could have ever worked. It was incredibly difficult for him to get around. His balance was shot and he couldn't get up steps with any ease. There weren't many options for people in his situation. But he was able to keep things going at home, and looked after our daughter Joan. But that too was difficult. There were times he had to tie her to a tree so she wouldn't wander off.

Joan was a godsend in so many ways. Not only was she a joy to us, but also she was a companion and help to her dad while I was off at work. When he tinkered with the car, for instance, Joan would be there to hand him the tools and as a result, she knows a lot about cars and can't be duped when she takes her vehicle to a garage for service. She's grateful to have had this very special opportunity to learn from her dad. They helped each other. He told a social worker that he missed not having been able to pick his daughter up and put her on his knee the way a regular dad could.

A Citizen Band radio became a very important part of his life. He made friends all over the place—Arnprior, Renfrew, out West, all around the world. If someone was in trouble, Gordon was the focal point. They would phone him and he would take it from there. Some of his best friends came from CB contacts. They would come to visit him. They all had funny names. Gordon, for instance was called the "good '49er" because he drove a 1949 Dodge which he kept in mint condition.

We traveled twice across Canada, but it was on our trip to Florida that Gordon came to appreciate how much more he could do if he used a wheelchair. We paid for our trips with the money accumulated on my unused sick leaves from work.

Polio surely affected my life too, but everything seemed to work out well. When I went back to teaching, the high school students were an inspiration. Furthermore, Joan and my husband appreciated me when I was home. The only worry was making sure we had enough money to get by. Luckily our medical expenses were covered by insurance.

Gordon had a stroke in 1986 but just before that he was so weak he couldn't straighten up when pulling himself up the steps from the garage. I would have to take his hand and walk him to his chair in the dining room. I guess that was post-polio syndrome. He was greatly helped by the CLSC who arranged for him to go to a day centre in Ottawa, which he enjoyed. After his stroke in 1986 he had to rely upon a wheelchair entirely. He died in 1987 at the age of 68, a Type A personality to the end, always striving for perfection in what he did and how he looked, never a hair out of place. Through it all we both became more patient and more tolerant individuals. It must have been hard for him to accept my participation in his striving for excellence. As for me, I don't think anyone at work knew I was coping with illness at home. I didn't complain nor ask for any special favours.

Gordon's polio helped me be the strong and independent person I am today. I became head of the French department in Shawville. I liked to get things done well. I'm a Type A personality too, I guess, and they all respected that, including the students. Many of them are still great friends and continue to bring joy to my life.

Finally, I would like to pay tribute to Bill Pirie, James Maclaren, and to the man who had the gravel pit, and the candy man, all of whom were good and faithful friends of Gordon's to the end. Gordon's sisters and my sisters were always there when we needed them too.

MR. & MRS. LEBLANC

Tell Me It is Important to Have Legs

[DANIÈLE LEBLANC]

THE DESIRE to make a testimonial about polio has echoed in me for a long time now. Both my parents had polio at a very young age and were affected by significant handicaps. Each had a leg whose knee would not straighten. I have always wanted to share my experiences.

An interesting irony of fate was that my parents both contracted polio in 1930. My father was born in 1930 and my mother in 1926. They were married when my mother was twenty-nine years old and my father twenty-five. In spite of their handicaps, they managed very well and I have only memories of two very autonomous parents. I have never wanted for anything or missed anything in life. You might consider that I was among the privileged, not only with my family, but also with my grandparents. I have one sister, four years my junior.

My mother was an intelligent, refined, and inquisitive woman. She was a pianist who also liked poetry that she recited by heart. She was interesting. My mother and my father liked to sit and talk, and they spoke well and had stimulating conversations full of great ideas.

My father hired people to take care of the interior and exterior of our home. Both my parents worked. My father was a businessman and my mother worked for the Quebec Society for Disabled Children. Both drove the family car without any adaptations. My father piloted planes, even parachuted, and sailed boats. They had nothing to prove, although everything was a challenge, especially for my father. I even think that having a family was a challenge. Someone had told them that there was no point in getting married because having children would be too difficult. Certain people tried to dissuade them from a family, but they thought that a family was important for a full and productive life.

Curiously, when I was young, I did not see anything abnormal about my parents. It took someone else to make me aware. When I was a teenager, a friend came over to the house and whispered in my ear, "What does your mother have?" "Polio," was my instant response. That was the only time that anyone had said anything about my parents.

They always had a good disposition. Perhaps as a family we were a little more organized and more active than other families who were more mobile. My mother often said, "Lucky that your father has a leg that doesn't work; otherwise imagine what else he could do. He never stops!" It never happened. That is why I became so upset during the latter years of his life when I saw his anger about having to slow down. He never really accepted his physical deterioration; it was different with my mother, who was well-prepared for aging.

I think that their attitudes had something to do with their positions in their families while growing up. Mother was the eldest of a family of seven. She was always very well respected within her family. There were sometimes looks of pity perhaps, but always at the same time an admiration.

For my father it was different because he was the youngest of three children from a middle-class family. I believe that they did not find it easy having a handicapped child. When I used to visit his family, I felt that we were all looked at differently and I imagined that my father lived with this "look" all his life. It seemed to have become a part of him to be judged differently from everyone else. He was a very strong man with a strong will, a great strength of character, and a very enterprising disposition. But at the same time, he reverberated with anger.

My father knew how to direct people. He was a leader. He never wanted help, except when it was absolutely necessary, and those were rare times. He would not ask but preferred that one guess at what he needed help with. This was confounding for us. We would have liked to know the code. His always refusing our help led us to feel that we were being rejected, as though we had no right to help him.

Personally, I never wanted to try any sports that my parents did not do. By the time I was an adult, I realised that if I did not ski, it was because my parents did not ski. In fact, I believe that when we follow the lives of our parents, then what they don't do, we don't do; others might, but we don't. As a child, I identified more with my mother. What mother liked, I liked; what she hated, I hated. So, when mother refused to fly with my father as pilot, I refused to go up too. She did not like riding on the sled behind the snowmobile, so neither did I. I am certain that this attitude prevented me from experiencing all that was available to me. On the other hand, when she later wanted to sail, I started to sail. This behaviour was not peculiar to our family or to polios.

My awareness with respect to my parents' condition grew in stages. As time went by, I found it difficult to look at them. I felt real sorrow to see them like that, especially my father, who experienced more and more difficulty walking with the passing years. In the winter, when he could not go to Florida, he was grouchy all the time. In the last years of his life I saw the huge effort he had to make just to get out of his armchair. Often I diverted my glance so that he would not see how much it hurt me to watch. After all, a daughter is someone who loves her father passionately. His pain and his struggle become her pain and her struggle. His condition deteriorated gradually and he knew that he had to face even more weakness and immobility.

I am sure that the condition of my parents had a deep impact on me. Today I work in the field of the arts. I do theatre and I know that I draw some of my inspiration from my family experiences, although I cannot define clearly exactly what they are. There were difficult times, but my parents were models of courage, will, and determination. Let us say that the unpleasant times, which are not easy to talk about, were there. I remember one day I was walking with my friend on the street when we came across a handicapped person and this friend said to me, "Me, I would rather be dead." He had not yet met my parents. I told myself, "Oh, my God! Wait until he sees my parents!" But I was able to face the situation. I understood his reaction and after that I did not worry.

As I grew up I could admit to some embarrassment, even a certain amount of shame. I deplored it, and when I felt this shame, I did not like myself, but it was there. I cannot deny it. It was as if the handicap of my parents reflected on me. I am tall and large-boned, and I have had the impression that others looked on me with pity as sometimes my parents through someone else's eyes may have evoked pity. There were times when people looked at me with a slight air of alarm. This was probably the same look my parents felt. When I was a teenager, if I thought that there was the least negative judgement regarding my parents, I intervened with vehemence.

My sister and I developed a particular degree of self-sufficiency at a younger age than most kids. As youngsters we carried the luggage and the bags when we traveled because our parents could not do it. On the other hand, we remained protected for a long time, as mother and father would have been in their families. But personally I would say that I have been truly autonomous only for the past few years. This may appear to be the opposite of what one might intuitively believe. The reality was that having parents handicapped by polio inevitably led to more attention and less autonomy. It was their habit to pay attention to everything, and they brooded over us, protected us, and packaged us as if we were wrapped up in ribbons. I now realize that as a consequence I have seen myself as handicapped too.

I am certain that my life would have been different if my parents had not contracted polio, but I do not know in which way. It would be as if I had been born in another country. I would be different, but how? Because of polio, my parents did not grow normally. As a very young person, I felt too large by the time I reached ten or eleven. I was taller than my sister and I was larger than my mother and my father. The house was too small for me, but for them it was better to be too small than too large. They had their way of organizing things that was not exactly appropriate for me. I was big and I felt somewhat choked.

Today I often feel an urge to leave and run because the rule at our house when we were very young was not to wander too far from home because neither of our parents could go out looking for us. We had to stay close to them. For the longest time I felt obligated to remain close to my parents even into adulthood.

Soon I will be leaving to go on a trip to India. It feels like I am going to the end of the world. I feel like I will have to walk. You see, when we were young, my parents made us walk. Everyone else took the bus to go to school, but I walked. They told me, "You have good legs, so walk." Today I am a good walker, as were my maternal grandparents who walked a lot.

One never spoke about polio in the family. I tried to speak about it in past years but it has always been a delicate subject, almost taboo. The last conversation that I did have with my father before he died was about this delicate subject and it was the first time that I succeeded in making him recognize that it was important to have legs. He always said that it did not matter whether one had legs or not, and that I was being superior with my belief that it mattered. My father said that it was all in the head and that's what counts. It is will, determination, ideas, and education. Not to have good legs was not so bad. He would add, "I could have had my legs and yet had an unhappy life. Therefore, young men and women, I repeat, you don't need legs to be happy."

It used to be that if I saw people who were having difficulties in life I would scorn them with "You see, my parents had trouble walking, and yet they lived well, functioned well, managed well, and you have all your limbs and your life does not seem to go well." I see now, only too clearly, that life is more complex than that. One cannot separate the physical from the moral. The most astonishing thing about all this was that my father continued to hold onto his ideas, whereas as I saw at any given moment in his life he had to make this incredible effort just to rise and although he called it will, I saw rage.

One time I said to him, "You cannot tell to me that it is not important to have a pair of good legs because when you tell me that, it is like you are telling me that my legs are useless. With these legs I can do a lot of things." He denied and denied, and then he turned himself toward me and said: "Yes, yes. They are important."

I felt relieved. God gave us fingers, hands, arms, and so forth, and all of them including our legs are significant. I like my legs. I am sure that he knew it, but Father did not want to admit it for fear of falling into self-pity for not having them. I would have liked to speak more about it at home, but my mother died young, and he had little time for these problems. To some extent, for a long time I thought that I could not walk. My father often asked us to go get a glass of water for him. One day when I was sitting on the sofa with my friend, I asked him if he could get me a glass of water. I never got up. Without realizing it, I was imitating my father.

I even selected my friends according to his need "to make myself useful". Over the last few years I have become aware that I have driven myself to become completely autonomous, to do everything myself, to take on more than I am able to do. At our home I did not do anything. Everything was done for me. My mother used to say, "We did not have children to be useful to us," and then she did everything herself. My sister and I were spoiled children. Today I like to meet people who have had polio. This gives me the opportunity and freedom to talk about it. Sometimes I discuss polio with my sister, but we do not think about it in the same way. Meeting people who have had polio brings me closer to my parents, in a roundabout way. Perhaps it is because my mother died as a young person. I would like to have seen what she would have been like as she aged.

Richard and André Decoste

The Need to Exorcise Memories

[Paul Decoste]

One may wonder what brought me to write this account of polio. It is a long time after the dust has settled, forty years, and yet I have felt the need to exorcise those memories (mine and those of my wife) which, to some degree, could return us to the obscure happier moments of our life as a couple. In 1994 I decided to write and publish the details of those unhappy events that marked our two lives forever in a book entitled *Le souffle des étoiles*, published in September 1995.

We lived in Chicoutimi after our marriage in 1951, more precisely, in the "Bassin", west of the city. We had two fine young sons, Richard and André, two-and-a-half years old and fourteen months old respectively, when on September 15, 1954, they were afflicted by that dreadful poliomyelitis. In just a few days following that fateful date, it was not possible to evaluate or estimate the extent of the after-effects that would persist, but their condition made us fear the worst. I saw, just like the doctors who came to visit them, that my two children could no longer flex or contract their muscles, and it was impossible to touch them without causing incredible pain in their arms and legs.

Local newspapers and radio described the symptoms clearly. It was already obvious that the virus had begun its work destroying our two children. Without being a doctor, I could clearly see that polio had invaded our home.

By mid-June 1954 we had been in a heat wave and some isolated cases were reported in the area. Then around August 15, after the visit of specialists delegated by the Ministry of Health, which included the famous Dr. Armand Frappier and representatives of the regional medical authority, it was announced that there was a possibility of a rather severe polio outbreak. The local press, however, kept silent about this, something that I never understood.

It was inconceivable what was going on. That same afternoon the first doctor told us, without even requesting more tests, that there was not much to do because they had severe tonsillitis and recommended that they be given aspirin. However, the media described the polio symptoms, and the sorry state of my children—strong fever, stiffness at the nape of the neck, difficulty breathing—and this made me suspect the worst. We were terribly upset with this total incompetence. I then called a doctor we knew. He insisted on a lumbar puncture at the hospital, which I refused because we were already well aware of the gravity of the situation that awaited us and of the possible consequences.

I also refused to have my children hospitalized because I knew that few specialized services were available at the Hôtel-Dieu in Chicoutimi. Also, I heard of parents complaining about the lack of suitable care for those already hospitalized during the height of the epidemic (in July particularly). So I did not see the benefit of transferring my children to the hospital only to confirm with a spinal tap what we already knew.

With the help of the competent doctor, my wife and I decided that the attention which we could give the boys at home would be more beneficial to them than at the small hospital, even though cases like these required trained personnel.

We undertook to give them frequent cold baths to lower their horrible fevers. Then, using a few but essential bits of furniture and accessories, we transformed their room into an "emergency room", which also became our permanent residence, hoping that it would be as temporary as possible. A young doctor whom I called Jean-Claude came every time he had the opportunity to bring us the help and support we needed.

After returning home, we consulted a chiropractor friend, who agreed to come to the house to give treatments; he provided invaluable suggestions. Later, continuing my never-ending quest to find something or someone that might help our children, I came across a "specialist" who began a series of electric shock treatments at his office. Not only was it very difficult to move and get the children there, it took only a few appointments before I began to detest his cavalier way of carrying out treatments and his general attitude in front of the children. So I decided to stop those visits. In my opinion, they did not provide anything worthwhile, and they caused pain and trauma to my little ones. Instead, we continued with the chiropractor.

During this time and up until mid-May 1955, there was no such thing as rehabilitation. I am not exaggerating when I say that there were no specialists available except for a young technician who, without adequate equipment, could do little despite all his good intentions. There was only one iron lung available in the Chicoutimi area for the acute cases with breathing problems.

Meanwhile, I met the representative to the House of Commons in Chicoutimi, Mr. V. Brassard, who had a small girl the same age as my son Richard. She was also a victim of poliomyelitis. He realized, like me, that there was a lack of organisation and specialized care. We formed an ad hoc committee with some other parents. Our first act was to go and borrow another iron lung from the military base at Bagotville, generously offered by the base authorities, who also arranged to have it brought to the hospital in Chicoutimi.

We had several meetings with the Mother Superior of the hospital in order to try to retain the services of more qualified doctors and obtain more adequate equipment. She did not seem to understand the importance of our movement and informed us that in any event these non-recurring expenses were not envisioned in the hospital budget. She did not believe that there was an epidemic in the area and could not see the urgency for such an expenditure. It was not long before she had to change her position, because a week later, we were told of the arrival of a doctor from Montreal whose mandate was to evaluate the severity of the "damage" and to recommend action. Following his recommendations was not that easy, however, because it was still not possible to obtain treatments locally, unless one wanted corrective orthopedic surgery which, in my opinion, was painful, expensive, and premature.

As for prescriptions to wear braces, which were sometimes absolutely necessary, one needed to go to the Laboratoire Auger in Quebec City. A specialist would come to take measurements, go back to Quebec City to manufacture the brace, and then return to Chicoutimi for fittings.

Towards the end of 1955 we finally saw the arrival of two physiotherapists, who came from Montreal Rehabilitation Institute. Neither spoke French. Communicating was rather difficult. Eager to take advantage of the new care available for my children, I invited the physiotherapists to come to the house to help with my two sons and to provide the treatments they gave to others at the hospital. Being bilingual myself, we were able to exchange ideas and quickly organize a treatment program for the children. They received physiotherapy once or twice a week which would have been more beneficial if it had been started earlier.

After learning that Dr. Gustave Gingras and Dr. Maurice Mongeau, both specialists from Montreal, were to visit Chicoutimi to study the many after-effects left on a good number of children, I scheduled a meeting with them. Dr. Gingras strongly recommended a stay at the Pasteur Hospital in Montreal, where they could give our children a more thorough examination with follow-up at the Montreal Rehabilitation Institute.

It was not easy to arrange suitable transportation, but we settled on the night train, eight in the evening to nine the following morning. The evaluation at the Rehabilitation Institute suggested that it was necessary to stay at the Pasteur where we believed that all the best care would be made available to them.

So it was with broken hearts that we left Richard and André to stay there for nearly six months, with only one visit per month allowed. From one visit to the next, I did not see any functional improvement and even less psychological. In the end, being away from Mom and Dad was too much for them, and they were very depressed.

Following a long conversation with Dr. Gingras, and having only one other option (going to the Atlanta Rehabilitation Center, in Georgia, in the United States), we decided to bring our sons home. My older brother offered to accompany them with my wife on the train, while I spent some time in Montreal learning the basic techniques of physiotherapy that would be particularly suitable for our sons.

On my return home, I plunged the boys into all kinds of prescribed exercises plus others that I invented myself which got results I am particularly proud of. I describe them in my book. In a significant way, the boys' general well-being greatly improved, as they regained their appetite, slept better, laughed and joked, all of which gave us the courage to continue, two hours every evening after my work.

Drs. Gingras and Mongeau explained to me later, during one of our monthly follow-ups at their office, that the father-son arrangement was very commendable and it showed very encouraging results for them. I humbly believe that all the years of these treatments contributed to keep them healthy and over time, brought them a better quality of life in every way. Each visit to Montreal did nothing more than confirm the continuing success of the treatments. This, I believe, was the best decision that I took from the beginning of our trials with the disease.

I owe an immense amount of gratitude to the personnel at the Pasteur and to all the other people who gave me training in the basics of physiotherapy and its elementary psychology. My persistence finally produced results: André managed to move on braces and crutches and Richard was doing very well in a wheelchair.

How does one describe this trial that could have taken the lives of our young sons? How did we as a young couple cope? Before the sad times, up to that eventful day on September 15, 1954, the possibilities for our sons were endless. We had dreamed of beautiful strong boys; they were born in good health. We organized our lives in order to bring to fruition all the dreams and hopes we held for our family, which included our daughter Josée who was born three years after the boys were diagnosed with polio.

I look at this sad truth, and what are we to make of it? Let ourselves be cut down? Cry and bemoan our fate? Damn this life which has left us so disabled? Not to smile any more at the two we love so much? No, that bespeaks little knowledge about us. Beyond this despair, only one thing remains to be done, and we have done it: we let go, to give body and soul so that our children can live fully, and to live a good life with us, to live in our love in bringing them everything we can possibly imagine, so that hope will smile again on their lives. It does not matter that they will not regain their robust capacities because, thanks to God, their intellects were not affected.

Through all the years of unrelenting suffering, of never-ending tears, my wife, in all her generosity and her strength, knew to continue to be who she was, which is her testament as a loving mother and devoted spouse full of love and compassion. She was the strength from which I drew the energy I needed to follow my assignments with my two small patients that tragic events had transformed into "small handicapped people" filled with love.

Fortunately, at the beginning of 1954 I had had the good sense to buy insurance which covered several infantile diseases including polio. During the years that followed, the insurance made it possible to deal with the huge hospital expenses and other related costs, which I would not have been able to meet, as was the case for many other parents with similar children. Owing to the fact that they were handicapped, the support would have continued to the end of their days.

Richard died at eighteen years old and André at thirty, both of pulmonary complications.

During that period when I was totally focused on my wife and my two children, my employer, Alcan, was very generous in giving me a prolonged leave. I still owe them a huge thank you and my heartfelt appreciation.

Not one day goes by without some reminder of the boys. Something points out all the joys which we shared together during what was their too short lives on this earth and which makes us appreciate them so much more, despite all the sorrow.

It is important to look at things in the context of the 1950s. One of the bitterest memories that I have was the obvious lack of hospital organisation, the impotence of medical service, particularly in our area, and finally the absence of will on the part of the medical and hospital authorities to cross the barrier that flagrantly separated care given to the wealthy compared to those less fortunate. The majority of the children affected by polio during the epidemic came from working-class families[1] who were without the resources to face costs inherent to the situation.

When I return to Chicoutimi, I notice that things have improved. The hospital is now equipped with the most beautiful and the most functional rehabilitation centre in the province.

Four

Teachers, Nurses, Doctors, and Volunteers

This section is dedicated to all those who helped make life in the hospital, at school or in the community, bearable. Some of us younger "polios" became so used to institutional living that we never wanted to go home. There were countless (but not all) doctors, nurses, physiotherapists, orderlies, and volunteers whose dedication to service and love for children shone through their professional work. Thorna Rountree, for instance, who taught me to read and write at the Children's Memorial Hospital and remained a lifelong friend until she died in 1993; beloved-by-all Jimmy who took me and countless others from the Ward L Hut to the main building to be x-rayed after falling out of bed for the umpteenth time while struggling to move; volunteer Miss Robinson, who gave me a cherished Scarlet O'Hara doll, and Miss Akagawa, a nurse whom I remember for her gentle kindness.

Andee Fortune remembers with affection Chief Physiotherapist, Miss Finley, who would pack some of the older kids into her car and take them for a drive or to her home. Another physio Doris Glover is also fondly remembered. More recently there was the late Anne-Marie van Daele who had trained in Belgium and Warm Springs. She followed her husband Paul from Belgium to Montreal where she taught and took on special polio cases. She was particularly helpful to Polio Quebec Association founder Sieglinde Stieda, and to Alice Westcott.

So the recollections of the polio years that follow, of a teacher and a nurse, are representative of ALL those who nurtured us young children, and some not so young, through difficult and confusing years.

–Sally Aitken

Even if You Are a Catholic, I Still Like You!

Mabel Wilmut Remembers
Teacher, 1950-1979

I WAS ASKED by the Montreal Catholic School Commission whether teaching at the Children's Memorial Hospital would interest me. They already had a teacher there and they needed a second one. I started in November 1950. I was only working six weeks when I came down with infectious hepatitis, along with most of the student nurses and some of the patients. I was off for two months.

Bedside teaching was quite a revelation. I was twenty-five and had never thought of teaching in a hospital. It was difficult finding my way around all those buildings at the Children's, and at the height of the polio epidemics. Joyce Wood was busy with the patients who had cerebral palsy. As a result, all the ward teaching was left to me. The polios were in an outside hut, Ward K. Another outside hut was devoted to those who had rheumatic fever, which was prevalent at the time. In the main hospital building there were the general, medical, and surgical wards. The only ward I didn't go into was the Isolation Ward. But the rheumatic fever and polio patients were the ones I got to know best because many of them were in the hospital for such a long time. I taught Grade 1 through Grade 11. If provincial exams had to be taken, we would arrange it. Finding a quiet room where they could write these exams was difficult.

What I remember most about the polio ward was the humidity caused by the hot packs. It was astounding. Beds were really crammed into that ward and all the hustle around the hot pack treatment made it difficult to keep a child's attention.

On the whole, the children welcomed being schooled in the hospital, because it was one thing they were familiar with. If I could turn up with the same book they had in school, it was like being a magician. At the beginning I used to have a supply of books at the hospital, but in later years I had to ask the parents to bring in their children's books.

I taught there for twelve years (1951-1963), making the move down to the building on Tupper in 1957. Having been away from the classroom for twelve years, I began to think I might be losing my norms, so I returned to a regular school for twelve years, and for my final four years' teaching I went back to the hospital (1975-1979). Nothing much had changed, except there was now a classroom big enough to accommodate a bed patient or two.

I taught the English Catholic patients. There was a teacher for French and then of course an English Protestant teacher, Margaret Ellis, who must have followed Thorna Rountree, then Sally Chapman and a succession of others. Finally it was decided to divide teaching responsibilities between wards rather than between religions. Noreen Tansey is the last Protestant teacher I remember. (Until 1998, Quebec's school system was a confessional one with separate Catholic and Protestant School Boards.)

I can remember a little child from the Maritimes who was forever in the hospital. He was a preschooler. I said to him, "You'll be in school next year." He thought I would be teaching him. I said that I wouldn't be teaching him because I was a Catholic and he wasn't. He stared at me for a long time and finally said, "Well, even if you are a Catholic, I still like you!"

The two students I remember very well are Daphne Dale-Bentley and Margot Senecal. I didn't teach Daphne because she wasn't a Catholic but she really impressed me by how well she had adapted to the severity of her polio. Her parents were so upset that they were quick to find fault with the hospital, but Daphne would reassure them that everything was fine. Margot, on the other hand, was a Catholic, and I taught her in her comings and goings to the hospital over a period of three years. I really got to know her. Margot's mother was forever after embarrassing me with her compliments about my role in her daughter's life.

Yes, I remember the great big orderly, Jimmy. All the children loved him, as they did another orderly whose name escapes me. He was so effective in calming distraught children.

Joyce Wood started teaching at the Children's Memorial Hospital in 1945. With her vast experience she became Special Ed Consultant at the Catholic School Commission in 1963.

Polio—"Infantile Paralysis" in My Time

Louise Oliver Remembers
Nurse 1932-1975

When I was about six years old, a young cousin died of infantile paralysis. The family lived on a farm so this was an isolated case. However, as I recall the family discussions, they were well aware of the seriousness of this disease and also the resulting crippling effects should a child survive. So I grew up quite aware of polio and its ramifications.

I trained to be a nurse at the Children's Memorial School of Nursing in 1929. I took a post-graduate course in surgery at Boston Children's Hospital, and worked in many capacities at the Children's Memorial, the Montreal Children's, the Lakeshore General, and the Lachine General Hospitals.

Around the year 1928 researchers discovered the presence of antibodies in the blood of patients who had an attack of polio. Thus was developed the "convalescent serum treatment" under the direction of Dr. P.N. MacDermott.

A doctor's concern for patients with paralytic respiratory complications led to the construction of the first respirator in the workshop of the Children's Memorial Hospital. Dr. Howard Mitchell directed Tom Wright's carpentry work. It was a crude machine by modern standards, but it worked and saved lives. One of these units was later shipped to the Nuffield Foundation in England from where, after modification, new models were built and sent to all parts of the world for emergency use. Every time the power goes off I remember the desperate struggle to keep a young polio patient alive.

The responsibility shouldered by the nurses in those epidemic years was phenomenal. In fact, the unsung heroes were the student nurses. It was they who carried the workload. At the Children's, under the direction of Madeleine Flanders (now Wilson), the students learned the underlying principles of child care: make the patient as comfortable as possible; prevent breakdown of the skin; maintain muscle tone; prevent deformity; offer good nutrition; and be morale boosters. Long-term-illness children were often frustrated by their lack of mobility or apparatus. It was a challenge to keep the children happy.

Madeleine Flanders was the finest supervisor I have ever known. She knew her nursing and the children and had a wealth of resources at her fingertips. No question was left unanswered. She always had time to listen.

Working closely with the doctors and nurses were the physiotherapists. Under the direction of Esther Asplit and her assistant Margaret Finlay, the polio patients' rehabilitation program was carried out. A special pool was constructed for hydrotherapy exercises.

I am sure it is difficult for doctors and nurses today to fully appreciate the enormity of challenges that faced the hospital staff during the first half of the twentieth century. However, I feel those who lived and worked then can be justifiably proud of their accomplishments and services in the polio saga.

Five

The Vaccine Story

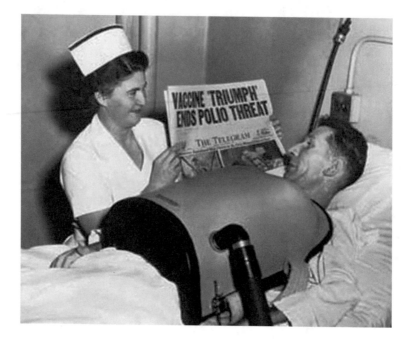

Headline, *The Telegram.*
Courtesy of Polio Canada.

The Beginning of the End: The Vaccine Story

SALLY AITKEN

The fear of polio galvanized broad segments of society to seek ways of preventing this crippling disease from ravaging their communities. Not knowing where the disease was coming from, people blamed everything from sick cats to dirty neighbourhood children, water, shared ice cream cones, and milk. Could mosquitoes or flies be transferring the poliovirus from fruit or garbage? Were swimming pools, rivers, lakes, creeks no longer safe? Even sniffing an infected rose bush from another province was suspected. The best protection against polio was to stay away from what was thought, rightly or wrongly, to be its cause. However, living in virtual isolation during the late summer and autumn months when polio was most likely to strike was just not possible. Increasingly, the traditional joys of summer were replaced by dread.

Drs. Salk and Sabin virtually stopped polio in its tracks. They were supported to a large extent by the unprecedented success of fundraising efforts inspired by U.S. President Franklin D. Roosevelt's personal and dedicated interest in polio. The National Foundation for Infantile Paralysis (NFIP) sprang from the Warm Springs Foundation. Warm Springs, developed by FDR at an existing resort in the state of Georgia, was a therapeutic rehabilitation camp for people with polio. The NFIP was one of the most successful voluntary health organizations in history. It raised enough money each year to pay hospital and rehabilitation costs for any polio patient who needed help in the United States, while sponsoring training programs for nurses and physical therapists and supporting the laboratory research that led to both the Salk and Sabin vaccines. It spent ten times as much on polio research as the tax-supported National Institute of Health, raising money from the vast reservoir of people whose vague desire to help the world had not been tapped previously.[1]

In 1938 when the NFIP shifted its fundraising focus away from Warm Springs and into every town in America, the Hollywood community became more involved. It was then that Los Angeles comedian Eddie Cantor started calling the January campaign "The March of Dimes", playing on the public's familiarity with the popular newsreel feature "The March of Time!" The first appeal was a spectacular success. "The Government of the United States darned near stopped functioning because we couldn't clear away enough dimes to find the official White House mail," complained the Chief of Mails at the White House.[2]

Fundraising was equally successful in Canada under the March of Dimes banner. But it wasn't until 1956 that the Quebec Command of the Royal Canadian Legion incorporated itself under the name "Quebec March of Dimes" in order to raise money for immunization clinics throughout the province. Due in great part to the efforts of Legion volunteers, more than two million immunizations of the Salk vaccine were administered between 1956 and 1961—sometimes as many as 10,000 in one evening, recalls Montreal legionnaire W.A. Rogers. In fact the eagerness to be immunized against this dreaded disease was so great, said Dr. Jean-Guy Bonnier (physician emeritus who worked in Ville LaSalle's public health department during the epidemic years), that people lined up along Boulevard LaSalle from LaSalle City Hall all the way to the Mercier Bridge.

Before the vaccine, however, research money went to testing nasal sprays and vitamin and hormone therapy, but all were proven to be virtually ineffective in preventing the epidemics of polio paralysis. The convalescent serum gave solace to those who felt something had to be done, anything; and it was used in the 1930s and into the 1940s. Physicians in some Canadian provinces were confident that paralytic polio could be prevented if a "convalescent serum" were administered early enough. Energy that could have been focused more constructively went uselessly into collecting and administering the blood of new polios for this serum. It was genuinely believed by some that if the public were educated to recognize the early signs of polio, prompt administration of the serum would prevent paralysis. Christopher Rutty's doctoral thesis on polio describes the pendulum of opinion on this serum. In the early 1940s it was finally abandoned as having no value.[3]

In 1936, two groups of U.S. investigators prepared vaccines from the brain and spinal cord of infected monkeys which were treated to inactivate the virus. Hundreds of people were vaccinated but some developed paralysis, presumed to be caused by a virus that had escaped inactivation. These experiments were promptly terminated and further progress in polio prophylactics awaited technical advances.[4] Throughout this period, polio prevention research was fueled by desperation, but Dr. Jonas Salk was convinced he was on the right track with his killed poliovirus theory. Dr. Albert Sabin's scepticism fell on deaf ears. In 1952, Salk tested his vaccine on himself and those working in Pittsburgh's Virus Research Lab, before injecting his inactivated poliovirus (IPV) into children at Pennsylvania's Polk State School and the D.T. Watson Home for Crippled Children. This pre-trial trial was very encouraging. So in January 1953, 161 people received one or another of several experimental vaccines from the University of Pittsburgh Viral Research Lab. The results were published in *The Journal of the American Medical Association* in March of that year. In April 1954, 650,000 children in 211 health districts of 44 U.S. states participated in a massive field trial of what by then became known as the Salk Polio vaccine.[5] In the Canadian trials, 12,456 received three doses of the vaccine and 12,320 were given the placebo, while a group of 14,976 were not inoculated.[6] Albert Sabin's live attenuated vaccine came onto the scene in 1960, having been widely tested in the U.S.S.R. and Poland. It is a vaccine that can be administered orally.

Three scientific breakthroughs underlay the development of these vaccines: the successful tissue culture of the poliovirus in non-nervous tissue by Enders, Weller, and Robbins in 1949, for which they were awarded the Nobel Prize for medicine in 1954;[7] the recognition that there were only three antigenically distinct strains of the virus; and the discovery that the administration of human immune serum globulin would prevent paralysis.[8]

In 1951, Canada played a pivotal role in the production and mass distribution of the virus for production of the vaccine. Dr. Joseph F. Morgan at the University of Toronto's Connaught Medical Research Laboratories had been using what he called Medium 199 for the study of cell nutrition in cancer research. He recommended this medium to his colleague and friend Dr. Arthur E. Franklin for growing the poliovirus. It worked,[9] ending Salk's need for animal serum, which consisted of anything from foreskins, miscarriages, or stillbirths. Salk had found that monkey testicles were effective, but Connaught's Medium 199—composed of over sixty ingredients[10]—gave Canada's Connaught Labs a major role in the production and dissemination of the Salk vaccine on both sides of the border. Without Connaught's Herculean efforts, there could never have been a trial, since no American laboratory had the experience or facilities to undertake such a financially risky project.[11]

Quick implementation of the vaccine program in Canada is attributed to the Honourable Paul Martin, Sr. In 1946 he had just been appointed to the U.N. when he got news that his son, eight-year old Paul, Jr., had contracted polio. It took almost a year before he fully recovered. Paul Martin, Sr. had had spinal meningitis (later referred to as polio) as a boy and his son's bout with polio reinforced his awareness of the need for a universally accessible response to polio. In 1953 the Canadian government funded the Connaught Lab's production of Medium 199 for the Salk polio vaccine. Martin made a deal with Maurice Duplessis that if he were to provide a new building for the Institute of Microbiology in Montreal, Ottawa would underwrite the cost of polio vaccine. And so it was thanks to Dr. Armand Frappier's leadership that the new labs were built and officially opened in 1954, allowing the Institut de

Microbiologie et d'Hygiène de l'Université de Montréal (which in 1975 became known as l'Institut Armand Frappier) to develop the means to mass produce the Salk vaccine. Dr. V. Pavilanis was in charge of this important project.

Of the many problems that had to be addressed, the most disturbing was that of the monkeys and the intestinal diseases (salmonella and shigella) that became apparent a few weeks after their arrival. Dr. Paul Marois had the complex task of caring for these monkeys and overseeing every aspect of their health during the work up to the final release of the Salk vaccine for public immunization in 1957. Doctors and technicians came from many countries to observe and learn the procedures being used by this laboratory in the production of the vaccine.[12] In the meantime, the University of Toronto's Connaught Lab's vaccine had become "a Canadian prestige item" and by June 1958 more than 5.5 million doses had been exported to Great Britain, while additional vaccine was shipped to a total of 44 countries.[13]

Martin would not authorize use of the vaccine in Canada until April 1955 after it had been approved in the United States. Two weeks following his press conference to announce the first experimental use of the vaccine in Canadian schools and after more than 100,000 children had been inoculated, there were some deaths in the U.S. attributed to the vaccine, and the program there was suspended. The immediate dilemma was to determine whether it was the vaccine itself that was at fault or a specific batch. Tormented by the thought that there might be a repeat of the 1954 epidemic if the program in Canada were discontinued, Martin hurriedly sought advice that convinced him that the problem was traceable to one of the U.S. pharmaceutical manufacturers. He concluded that the Connaught lab in Toronto was "clean" and that immunization programs must proceed at full speed. That was the summer of 1955. Said Martin, "When I look back on the achievement of the health program, I see it as one of the major contributions of my public life. ... I see this most keenly in my own family. The Salk vaccine conquered poliomyelitis and saved the lives of youngsters. Both my son Paul and I had suffered from polio as children and I knew as well as most, the importance of the vaccine that was combating it."[14]

So it was in 1955 that children throughout North America were injected with the Salk vaccine. This was replaced by the live Sabin Oral Polio Vaccine (OPV) in 1962. It had been widely tested in the U.S.S.R. and Poland as far back as 1956, but it wasn't until March 6, 1962 that Connaught's trivalent (containing all three strains of polio) was licensed in Canada, the first such type to be licensed internationally.[15] According to V. Pavilanis of the Institut de Microbiologie et d'Hygiène, the inactivated poliovirus vaccine (Salk) had a preventive action in Canada of 95 percent. But only 70 percent of the

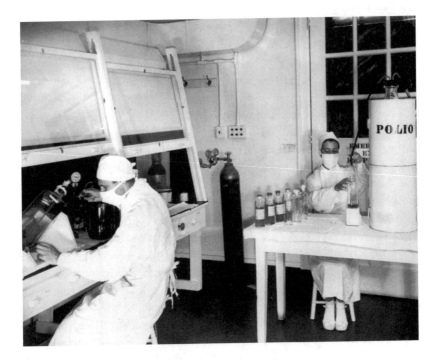

Large scale production of poliovirus fluids at Connaught Medical
Research Laboratories, University of Toronto for the
Salk Vaccine Field Trial, 1954.
Aventis Pasteur Limited Archives.

population was being reached, and the incidence of polio among those not vaccinated was in the range of 27.1 per 100,000.[16]

On the other hand, the Sabin vaccine (live virus) conveyed indirect immunity to the population at large. Therein lay the appeal of the oral Sabin vaccine. Conversely, on very rare occasions fecal infection from the diaper of a recently-vaccinated infant transferred the poliovirus to a care giver who was not immune. (At least three current members of Polio Quebec got polio this way.) Needless to say this wholly unexpected outcome, although rare, attracted press coverage, which lead to suspicion and rejection of the vaccine by some people. Statistically, the incidence of contracting polio this way is 1 in 2.5 million, which is no longer acceptable in countries that are rid of the wild virus. Consequently, over a period of a few years, all Canadian provinces have gone back to the inactivated Salk polio vaccine (IPV).

A brief description of these two vaccines from the World Health Organization's (WHO) book, Polio: The Beginning of the End (pages 7-8) helps one to understand why in polio-free countries Salk's dead vaccine is now preferred, why in countries where the wild virus still persists that continued use of the Sabin vaccine makes sense, and why our government continues to invest millions of dollars annually in immunization programs and will continue doing so until polio, like smallpox, has been definitively eradicated.

We will never be able to put to rest completely the doubts some people have about vaccinations, polio included.[17] Whether the fear stems from possible Simian (monkey) virus 40 (SV40) contamination of the vaccine[18] or from the potential of future ailments from having been subjected to a vaccine, it is important to note that by 1962 (following the discovery of SV40 contamination in some batches of polio vaccines in 1960), vaccines have been completely free of SV40.[19] What is more, the present use of the killed virus vaccine in Canada removes the risk of contracting polio indirectly from a recently vaccinated individual.

It was hoped that by the year 2000 polio, like smallpox, would be a disease of the past. The goal for worldwide eradication of this dreaded disease was set by the World Health Organization in 1988, but because of local conflicts that have thwarted many immunization programs, the target date for total polio eradication has been moved forward to the year 2005. It might well be achieved, given impressive cooperation from a coalition that includes Rotary International, UNICEF, the U.S.A., Japan, the U.K., Denmark, Canada, Australia, Germany and many other countries. Even manufacturers have donated vaccine to the cause. However, the most important partners are the polio-endemic countries themselves. Rotary International spearheaded the polio eradication objective prior to 1988—in 1985 in fact—when it launched its twenty-year

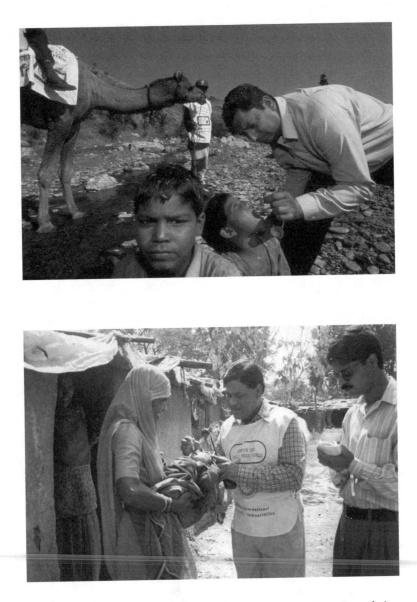

(top) India, 1998. National Immunization Days. 100,000 Rotarians, their families, friends, co-workers and the Indian government immunized 130 million children in one day. *Photo by Marcus Oleniuk.*
(bottom) India, 1999. Indian Rotarian giving Polio vaccine to a village infant outside family hut.
Rotary International Image Library.

crusade to help immunize every child against polio. Although this was a monumental task for a community-based organization, it is being over-whelmingly successful, providing major funding and mobilizing literally millions of volunteers worldwide. Their program became known as PolioPlus and accounts of its progress can be read monthly in Rotary International's Rotarian Magazine. Rotarians in Canada gave $12 million Canadian during the original PolioPlus campaign from 1985 to 1989. Of this amount, $746,445 came from the Province of Quebec. Members of these four clubs personally donated $400,000. Several Rotarians from Canada served as volunteers of National Immunization Days, commonly referred to as NIDs. Canadian Rotarians have contributed a total of US$457,249 to the PolioPlus Partners program since the program's inception in November 1995. PolioPlus was set up to provide tools of immunization for National Immunization Days in developing countries. Those tools include everything that will bring children to the immunization sites—publicity materials (pamphlets, posters, banners, billboards), T-shirts to identify volunteers, audio equipment, and lollipops to reward children. Funds are also used to purchase vaccine carriers, bicycles, and lab equipment.

In May 1998 the Canadian International Development Agency committed $10 million Canadian a year for five years to combat polio and other childhood diseases. On February 3, 1999, Bill Huntley, past Rotary International president and incoming Rotary Foundation chairman, presented the Polio Eradication Champion Award to Prime Minister Jean Chrétien in recognition of Canada's commitment to polio eradication in the poorest countries of Africa and Asia.

Dr. John Carsley of the Montreal-Centre Regional Public Health Department, while keeping tight control over the administration of vaccines in general, urges anyone who is sceptical about the polio vaccine to talk to their family physician, pediatrician, or public health department about their concern. "And above all," he says, "don't postpone or forego vaccines important to you or your children's health."

ORAL VERSUS INJECTIBLE / LIVE VERSUS KILLED VIRUS VACCINES

Oral polio vaccine works by inducing not only serum immunity but also secretory immunity, particularly inside the intestines, the primary site for poliovirus multiplication. As well as inducing individual protection against polio, OPV also limits the multiplication of "wild" (naturally occurring) virus inside the gut. Immunization with OPV therefore creates an effective barrier against circulation of wild poliovirus by reducing fecal excretion of the virus.

However, a "helpful" outcome of immunization with OPV is the short-term shedding of vaccine virus in the stools of recently immunized children. In

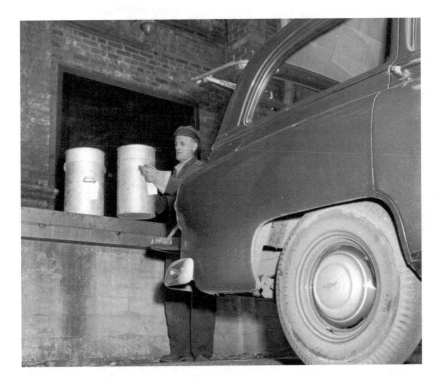

Loading bulk poliovirus fluids for shipment from Connaught Medical Research
Laboratories to Parke Davis (Detroit) or Eli Lilly (Indianapolis)
for final processing into Salk vaccine for NFIP field trial, 1954.
Aventis Pasteur Limited Archives.

areas where hygiene and sanitation are poor—and the incidence of polio is highest—immunization with OPV can result in the passive immunization of close contacts through the spread of vaccine virus shed in stools.

An added advantage of OPV is that it does not have to be administered by a trained health worker and, unlike most other vaccines, does not require sterile injection equipment. It is also relatively inexpensive, a major consideration when governments have to purchase massive quantities of vaccine for use in national immunization days. For these reasons OPV is the vaccine of choice for the eradication of polio. The downside is that, although OPV is safe and effective, the live attenuated vaccine virus can cause paralysis, although very rarely, either in the vaccinated child or in a close contact (about one in every 2.5 million doses administered).

Inactivated polio vaccine works by producing protective antibodies in the blood, thus preventing the spread of the poliovirus to the central nervous system. However, it induces only very low-level immunity to poliovirus inside the gut. As a result, it provides individual protection against polio paralysis but only marginally reduces the spread of the wild poliovirus. In a person immunized with IPV, the wild virus can still multiply inside the intestines and be shed in the stools. Because of this, IPV is only used to eradicate polio in countries that are polio-free.

The disadvantages of IPV include the price (over five times the cost of OPV), the cost of the needle and syringe, and the need for trained health workers to administer the vaccine using sterile injection procedures. However, IPV does not carry the risk of paralysis associated with OPV, and a number of industrialized countries (Canada included) have implemented, or are now considering implementing, a combined IPV/OPV schedule in their routine immunization program. The aim is to reduce the risk of vaccine-associated polio while maintaining the benefits of the high levels of intestinal immunity produced by OPV.

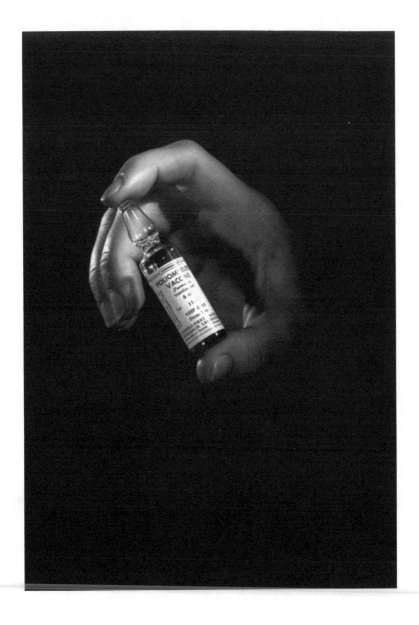

Aventis Pasteur Limited Archives.

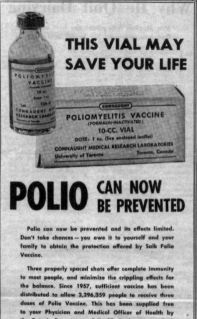

THIS VIAL MAY SAVE YOUR LIFE

POLIOMYELITIS VACCINE
(FORMALIN-INACTIVATED)
10-CC. VIAL
DOSE: 1 cc. (See enclosed leaflet)
CONNAUGHT MEDICAL RESEARCH LABORATORIES
University of Toronto   Toronto, Canada

POLIO CAN NOW BE PREVENTED

Polio can now be prevented and its effects limited.
Don't take chances — you owe it to yourself and your
family to obtain the protection offered by Salk Polio
Vaccine.

Three properly spaced shots offer complete immunity
to most people, and minimize the crippling effects for
the balance. Since 1957, sufficient vaccine has been
distributed to allow 2,296,359 people to receive three
doses of Polio Vaccine. This has been supplied free
to your Physician and Medical Officer of Health by
the Ontario Department of Health. In the same period,
the number of cases of Polio has shown a sharp
decline attributed mainly to the intensive vaccination
program.

Now is the time to act — summer and fall are the
main polio seasons. Arrange your family's vaccination
program today.

FROM INFANCY TO 40 YEARS

The most critical ages for Polio are from infancy
to 40 years. It is most important for everyone in these
age groups to receive three properly spaced Polio
Vaccine shots. Consult your local physician or Medical
Officer of Health.

ONTARIO DEPARTMENT OF HEALTH

ONTARIO

HON. MATTHEW B. DYMOND, M.D.
Minister

Courtesy of Christopher Rutty.

End Notes

SECTION ONE

The History of Poliomyelitis

1 W.J. McCormick, "Clinical Study of the Poliomyelitis and Encephalitis Epidemic in Western America and Canada in 1941", *L'Union médicale du Canada*, No. 71, 1942, p. 138.

2 C. J. Rutty, *Poliomyelitis in Canada*, 1927-1962, doctoral thesis, History Department, University of Toronto, 1995, p. 33.

3 *Taber's Encyclopedic Medical Dictionary* (11th ed.), 1970, p. 77. Cited in Edmund Sass, *Polio's Legacy*, University Press of America, 1996, p. 1.

4 Gustave Charest, "La poliomyélite antérieure aiguë ou paralysie infantile", *L'Union médicale du Canada*, No. 83, 1954, p. 1131.

5 F. Yergeau, "Poliomyélite", *L'Union médicale du Canada*, No. 47, 1918, p. 38.

6 P. Lépine, "Le Problème de la poliomyélite et l'orientation des recherches", *L'Union médicale du Canada*, No. 78, 1949, p. 8.

7 Sass, p. 3.

8 Rutty, pp. 225-227, 285-291.

9 Jean Saucier, "Le traitement de la poliomyélite par la méthode de Sister Kenny", *L'Union médicale du Canada*, No. 71, 1942, p. 595.

10 Rutty, p. 41.

11 Rutty, p. 84.

12 Rutty, p. 150.

13 Letter from Canadian Association of Physiotherapists, September 14, 1946. Ste. Justine Hospital Administrative Archives, Montreal.

14 Ste. Justine Hospital Administrative Archives.

15 Letter from Dr. Jean Saucier, February 17, 1939. Ste. Justine Hospital Administrative Archives.

16 Rutty, p. 240.

17 Charest, p. 52.

18 Rutty, p. 376.

19 Rutty, p. 114.

20 Charest, p. 1132.

21 Annual Report of the Quebec Minister of Health and Welfare, 1959.

22 Rutty, p. 397.

23 Rutty, p. 250.

Sister Kenny

24 Lauro S. Halstead, "Post-Polio Syndrome", *Scientific American*, April 1998, p. 43.

25 Victor Cohn, *Sister Kenny: The Woman Who Challenged the Doctors,* Burns & MacEachern, 1975, p. 20.

26 Cohn, pp. 40-41.

27 Cohn, pp. 72-82.

28 Cohn, p. 129.

29 C. J. Rutty, *Poliomyelitis in Canada, 1927-1962,* doctoral thesis, History Department, University of Toronto, 1995, pp. 146-149.

30 J.B. Scriver, *The Montreal Children's Hospital: Years of Growth,* McGill-Queen's University Press, p. 111.

31 Rutty, p. 155.

Post-Polio Syndrome

32 T.J. John, "The Final Stages of the Global Eradication of Polio", *New England Journal of Medicine,* 2000, vol. 343, pp. 806-807.

33 P.E. Parsons, letter in *New England Journal of Medicine,* 1991, vol. 325, p. 1108.

34 B. Jubelt, N.R. Cashman, "Neurological Manifestations of the Post-Polio Syndrome", *CRC Critical Reviews in Neurobiology,* 1987, vol. 3, pp. 199-220.

35 T.L. Munsat, "Poliomyelitis: New Problems with an Old Disease", *New England Journal of Medicine,* 1991, vol. 324, pp. 1206-1207.

36 "Post-Polio Syndrome: Identifying Best Practices in Diagnosis and Care". March of Dimes Birth Defects Foundation (White Plains, NY, www.modimes.org) 2001.

37 L.S. Halstead, "Post-Polio Syndrome: Definition of an Elusive Concept", in T.L. Munsat, ed., *Post-Polio Syndrome,* Butterworth-Heinemann, 1991, pp. 23-38.

38. L.S. Halstead, C.D. Rossi, "Post-Polio Syndrome: Clinical Experience with 132 Consecutive Outpatients", in L.S. Halstead, D.O. Wiechers, eds., *Research and Clinical Aspects of the Late Effects of Poliomyelitis,* March of Dimes Birth Defects Foundation, 1987, pp. 13-26.

39 Jubelt and Cashman, pp. 199-220.

40 M.B. Codd, D.W. Mulder, L.T. Kurland, C.M. Beard, W.M. O'Fallon, "Poliomyelitis in Rochester, Minnesota, 1935-1955: Epidemiology and Long-Term Sequelae. A Preliminary Report", in L.S. Halstead, D.O. Wiechers, eds. *Late Effects of Poliomyelitis,* Symposia Foundation (Miami, FL), 1985, pp. 121-134.

41 J.L. Speier, R.R. Owen, M. Knapp, J.K. Canine, "Occurrence of Post-Polio Sequelae in an Epidemic Population", in Halstead and Wiechers, 1987, pp. 39-48.

42 A.J. Windebank, J.R. Daube, W.J. Litchy, M. Codd, E.Y.S. Chao, L.T. Kurland, R. Iverson, "Late Sequelae of Paralytic Poliomyelitis in Olmsted County, Minnesota", in Halstead and Wiechers, 1987, pp. 27-38.

43 A.J. Windebank, W.J. Litchy, J.R. Daube, L.T. Kurland, M.B. Codd, R. Iverson, "Late Effects of Paralytic Poliomyelitis in Olmsted County, Minnesota", *Neurology,* 1991, vol. 41, pp. 501-507.

44 J. Ramlow, M. Alexander, R. LaPorte, C. Kaufman, L. Kuller, "Epidemiology

of the Post-Polio Syndrome", *American Journal of Epidemiology*, 1992, vol. 136, pp. 769-786.

45 F. Lonnberg, M. Madsen, "Late Onset Polio Sequelae in Denmark", *Scandinavian Journal of Rehabilitation Medicine Supplement*, 1993, vol. 28, pp. 17-23.

46 M.C. Dalakas, G. Elder, M. Hallett, J. Ravits, M. Baker, N. Papadopoulos, P. Albrecht, J. Sever, "A Long-Term Follow-Up Study of Patients with Post-Poliomyelitis Neuromuscular Symptoms", *New England Journal of Medicine*, 1986, vol. 31, pp. 959-963.

47 D.A. Trojan, N.R. Cashman, *Current Trends in Post-Poliomyelitis Syndrome, Milestone Medical Communications* (a division of Ruder-Finn), 1996, pp. 27-30.

48 G. Grimby, A.L. Thoren-Jonsson, "Disability in Poliomyelitis Sequelae", *Physical Therapy*, 1994, vol. 74, pp. 415-424.

49 Jubelt and Cashman, pp. 199-220.

50 D.O. Wiechers, S.L. Hubbell, "Late Changes in the Motor Unit after Acute Poliomyelitis", *Muscle and Nerve*, 1981, vol. 4, pp. 524-528.

51 D.O. Wiechers, "New Concepts of the Reinnervated Motor Unit Revealed by Vaccine-Associated Poliomyelitis", *Muscle and Nerve*, 1988, vol. 11, pp. 356-364.

52 C. Coers, A.L. Wolf, *Special Pathology of the Intramuscular Nerves and Nerve Endings*. Innervation of Muscle. Biopsy Study, Charles C. Thomas Publishing, 1959, pp. 64-66.

53 Jubelt and Cashman, pp. 199-220.

54 D.A. Trojan, N.R. Cashman, "Pathophysiology and Diagnosis of Post-Polio Syndrome", *NeuroRehabilitation*, 1997, vol. 8, pp. 83-92.

55 R.L. Bennett, G.C. Knowlton, "Overwork Weakness in Partially Denervated Skeletal Muscle", *Clinical Orthopaedics*, 1958, vol. 12, pp. 22-29.

56 G.C. Knowlton, R.L. Bennett, "Overwork", *Archives of Physical Medicine and Rehabilitation*, 1957, vol. 38, pp. 18-20.

57 J. Perry, G. Barnes, J.K. Gronley, "The Post-Polio Syndrom: An Overuse Phenomenon", *Clinical Orthopaedics and Related Research*, 1988, vol. 233, pp. 145-162.

58 E.A. Muller, "Influence of Training and of Inactivity on Muscle Strength", *Archives of Physical Medicine and Rehabilitation*, 1970, vol. 51, pp. 449-462.

59 Jubelt and Cashman, pp. 199-220.

60 A.J. McComas, C. Quartly, R.C. Griggs, "Early and Late Losses of Motor Units after Poliomyelitis", *Brain*, 1997, vol. 120, pp. 1415-1421.

61 Halstead and Rossi, 1987, pp. 13-26.

62 Windebank, Daube, Litchy, Codd, Chao, Kurland, Iverson, pp. 27-38.

63 Windebank, Litchy, Daube, Kurland, Codd, Iverson, pp. 501-507.

64 Ramlow, Alexander, LaPorte, Kaufman, Kuller, pp. 769-786.

65 J. Klingman, H. Chu, M. Corgiat, J. Perry, "Functional Recovery: A Major Risk Factor for the Development of Postpoliomyelitis Muscular Atrophy", *Archives of Neurology*, 1988, vol. 45, pp. 645-647.

66 D.A. Trojan, N.R. Cashman, S. Shapiro, C. Tansey, J.M. Esdaile, "Predictive

Factors for Post-Poliomyelitis Syndrome", *Archives of Physical Medicine and Rehabilitation*, 1994, vol. 75, pp. 770-777.

67 Klingman, Chu, Corgiat, Perry, pp. 645-647.

68 Trojan, Cashman, pp. 83-92.

69 N.R.Cashman, R. Maselli, R.I. Wollman, R. Ross, R. Simon, J.P. Antel, "Late Denervation in Patients with Antecedent Paralytic Poliomyelitis", *New England Journal of Medicine*, 1987, vol. 317, pp. 7-12.

70 Trojan, Cashman, pp. 83-92.

71 A.C. Gawne, L. S. Halstead, "Post-Polio Syndrome: Pathophysiology and Clinical Management", *Critical Reviews in Physical and Rehabilitation Medicine*, 1995, vol. 7, pp. 147-188.

72 D.A. Trojan, L. Finch, "Management of Post-Polio Syndrome", *Neuro-Rehabilitation*, 1997, vol. 8, pp. 93-105.

73 P. E. Peach, S. Olejnik, "Post-Polio Sequelae: Effect of Treatment and Noncompliance on Post-Polio Sequelae", *Orthopaedics*, 1991, vol. 14, pp. 1199-1203.

74 Gawne and Halstead, pp. 147-188.

75 Trojan and Finch, pp. 93-105.

76 R.M. Feldman, C.L. Soskolne, "The Use of Non-Fatiguing Strengthening Exercises in Post-Polio Syndrome", in Halstead and Wiechers, 1987, pp. 335-341.

77 D.R. Jones, J. Speier, K. Canine, R. Owen, G.A. Stull, "Cardiorespiratory Responses to Aerobic Training by Patients with Postpoliomyelitis Sequelae", *Journal of the American Medical Association*, 1989, vol. 261, pp. 3255-3258.

78 J.C. Agre, A.A. Rodriguez, "Muscular Function in Late Polio and the Role of Exercise in Post-Polio Patients", *NeuroRehabilitation*, 1997, vol. 8, pp. 107-118.

79 W.P. Waring, F. Maynard, W. Grady, R. Grady, C. Boyles, "Influences of Appropriate Lower Extremity Orthotic Management on Ambulation, Pain, and Fatigue in a Post-Polio Population", *Archives of Physical Medicine and Rehabilitation*, 1989, vol. 70, pp. 371-375.

SECTION TWO

Dr. Herta Guttman

1 For some reason none of the restrictions that applied to many other patients in those days were applied to Herta. She was not put into isolation and her mother was able to stay with her. At the Children's Memorial it was isolation and an hour a week visiting on Sundays only.

2 The Post-Polio Clinic at the Montreal Neurological Institute and Hospital was not in place until 1988, by which time Dr. Cashman had organized a multi-disciplinary team of experts for the growing number of old polios who were seeking help with their new symptoms.

Elizabeth Goodfellow
1 Knatchbull-Hugessen, Kenneth Wyndham, "Jeunesse and Other Poems", 1944.

From the Bombed-out Hospital in Stettin—Sieglinde Stieda
1 Because Mme Grégoire had a science background, she was able to understand all the articles brought to her by Sieglinde. She damaged her shoulder muscles even further because of all the telephone calls she took.

2 In *Research and Clinical Aspects of the Late Effects of Poliomyelitis*, eds. Lauro S. Halstead and David O. Wickers. (From *Birth Defects*: Original Article Series, Vol. 3, number 4, 1987, pages 173-181).

3 See *Eat Right for Your Type*, by Peter d'Adamo.

4 Frances Cooke McGregor's writings (and telephone conversation) were helpful to Sieglinde, referring her to *The Harvard Law Review* No. 100 that deals with the legal ramifications of facial disfigurement.

SECTION THREE

Michel Robitaille
1 The March of Dimes was officially incorporated in 1951, an American initiative resulting from the extraordinarily successful fundraising efforts triggered by Franklin D. Roosevelt, who had had his personal struggle with polio. It was Eddie Cantor who coined the slogan "March of Dimes". In 1955 the Salk vaccine was discovered in part through research funded by the March of Dimes and with significant assistance from the Connaught Laboratory in Toronto.

2 Bell Canada made it possible for Michel to keep up with his classmates by connecting him at home in bed to the classroom at the School for Crippled Children by means of a loudspeaker and a microphone. Michel was the first to benefit from the Home Schooling Service offered by Bell.

Neil Compton
1 Dr. J. Cyril Flanagan is specially remembered by Gabriel (Compton) Baugniet as being their Robin Hood at the time.

Richard and André Decoste
1 Ed. note: This was an individual perception; polio was prevalent in all socio-economic groups.

Section Five

The Beginning of the End—The Vaccine Story

1 Jane S. Smith, *Patenting the Sun: Polio and the Salk Vaccine*, 1982, pp. 64 - 65.

2 Smith, p. 73.

3 C.J. Rutty, *Poliomyelitis in Canada*, 1927-1962, doctoral thesis, History Department, University of Toronto, 1995, p. 70.

4 Dr. Fred Robbins, "The quest for a vaccine," p. 14. Article in WHO's 48th Year, No. 1, 1995

5 Smith, p. 177.

6 Rutty, p. 325.

7 Rutty, p. 335.

8 Dr. Larry I. Lutwick, "Warts on the Poliosaur Bones: The Successes and Failures of Poliomyelitis Vaccines." *Medscape*. June 26, 1997.

9 C.J. Rutty, "40 Years", *Abilities Magazine*, Summer 1994, p. 26.

10 Smith, p. 130.

11 Smith, p. 177.

12 Dr. Armand Frappier, *Un rêve, une lutte*. Autobiographie, Presses de l'Université du Québec, 1992, p. 193.

13 Rutty, p. 347.

14 The Hon. Paul Martin, Sr., *A Very Public Life*. Deneau Publishers, 1983,1985.

15 Rutty, p. 356.

16 V. Pavilanis, "Problèmes de la vaccination antipoliomyélitique." *L'Union médicale du Canada*, 93 : 1964, p.1303–06.

17 Michael A. Prytuland. "No Vaccines for my Kids!" *Alive Magazine* #155, p. 15.

18 Elizabeth Pennisi, "Monkey Virus DNA Found in Rare Human Cancers." *Science*, vol. 275, February 7, 1997.

19 Dr. Robert Pless, VAAE Surveillance Section, Division of Immunization. FAX Memo to provincial epidemiologists/Immunization. February 24, 1997.

Appendix

Polio Canada (National)
10 Overlea Blvd
Toronto, ON
M4H 1A4
Tel. 800 480 5903 x257
Fax 416 426 1920
info@poliocanada.com
www.poliocanada.com

NEWFOUNDLAND
Newfoundland Society for the Physically Disabled
Southcott Hall #712
100 Forest Road
St. John's, NF
A1A 1E5
Tel: (709) 754 1399
Fax: (709) 754 1398
brentsmith@nspd.nf.ca
www.nspd.nf.ca

Polio Newfoundland
Carolyn Few
Tel. (709) 739-4299
cfew@nfld.com

PRINCE EDWARD ISLAND
Polio PEI
47 Westwood Crescent
Charlottetown, PEI
C1A 8X4
Tel: (902) 566 4518
sdpate@islandtelecom.com

NOVA SCOTIA
Abilities Foundation of Nova Scotia
Mrs. Ginny Phillips, Program Committee Chairperson
3670 Kempt Road
Halifax, NS
B3K 4X8

Tel: (902) 453 6000
Fax: (902) 454 6121
admin@abilitiesfoundation.ns.ca
www.abilitiesfoundation.ns.ca

NEW BRUNSWICK
Polio New Brunswick
268 Montreal Avenue
St. John, NB
E2M 3K6
Tel: (560) 635 8932
peterhef@nbnet.nb.ca

Polio Northern New Brunswick
1436 St. Mary Ave.
Bathurst, NB
E2A 2E3
Tel: (506) 548 1919
cggl@nbnet.nb.ca

New Brunswick Easter Seal March of Dimes
Mrs June Hooper, Executive Director
65 Brunswick Street
Fredericton, NB
E3B 1G5
Tel: (506) 458 8739
Fax: (506) 457 2863
jehooper@nb.aibn.com
esmodnb@nb.aibn.com
http://www.nbeastersealmarchofdimes.ca

QUEBEC
Polio Quebec Association
P.O. Box 1030
Station B
Montreal, QC
H3B 3K5
Tel: 1 800 263 1969; (514) 866 1969
Fax: (514) 866 6124
polioquebec@hotmail.com
www.polioquebec.org

ONTARIO
Post-Polio Program
c/o Ontario March of Dimes
10 Overlea Blvd.
Toronto, ON
M4H 1A4
Tel: 1-800 263 3463 or (416) 425 3463
Fax: (416) 425 1920
www.dimes.on.ca
polio@dimes.on.ca

MANITOBA
Society for Manitobans with Disabilities
Tom Kean, President and CEO
825 Sherbrook St.
Winnipeg, MB
R3A 1M5
Tel: (204) 975 3036
Fax: (204) 975 3011
tkean@smd.mb.ca
www.smd-services.com

Post-Polio Network (Manitoba) Inc.
c/o SMD Self-Help Clearinghouse
825 Sherbrook St.
Winnipeg, MB
R3A 1M5
Tel: (204) 772 6979
www.smd-clearinghouse.com

SASKATCHEWAN
Saskatchewan Awareness of Post-Polio
2310 Louise Avenue
Saskatoon, SK
S7J 2C7
Tel: (306) 343 0225
www.sfn.saskatoon.sk.ca/health/polio/

Polio Regina Inc.
4264 Wascana Ridge
Regina, SK
S4N 2T2
(306) 761-1020
bubbiecarole@accesscomm.ca

ALBERTA
Easter Seals March of Dimes
Susan Law, Executive Director
103, 811 Manning Rd NE
Calgary, AB
T2E 7L4
Tel. (403) 235 5662
Fax: (403) 248 1716
1(877) 732 7857 Toll Free
susan@esmod.ab.ca
www.esmod.ab.ca

Southern Alberta Post Polio Support Society
#7 - 11 St. NE
Calgary, AL
T2E 4Z2
Tel: (403) 265 5041
Fax: (403) 265 0162
sappss@shaw.ca

Wildrose Polio Support Society
Pat Laird
c/o CPA (Alberta)
305 Hys Centre
11010 - 101 St.
Edmonton, AB   T5H 4B9
Tel. (780) 992-0969
wpss_edm@hotmail.com

BRITISH COLUMBIA
Post Polio Awareness and Support Society of British Columbia
#2-2630 Ross Lane
Victoria, BC
V8T 5L5
Tel. (250) 477-8244
Fax: (250) 477-8287
ppass@ppass.bc.ca
www.ppass.bc.ca

NORTHWEST TERRITORIES
NWT Council of Persons with Disabilities
5014 47th Street
Yellowknife, NWT
X1A 1M1

Tel. 1-800-491-8885 or (867) 873-8230
Fax. (867) 873-4124
dbaptiste@nt.sympatico.ca

U.S.A.
International Polio Network
Gazette International Networking Institute (GINI)
4207 Lindell Blvd. #110
St. Louis, MO
63108-2915
Tel: (314) 534 0475
Fax: (314) 534 5070
Contact: Joan Headley
gini_intl@msn.com
www.post-polio.org

POST-POLIO ASSESSMENT CENTRES, CLINICS,
AND HEALTH PROFESSIONALS

NOVA SCOTIA
Dr. Benstead, Neurologist
The Halifax Infirmary
3rd Floor, Suite 3828
1796 Summer Street
Halifax, NS
B3H 3A7
Tel: (902) 473 2700

NEW BRUNSWICK
Dr. Colleen O'Connell
Stan Cassidy Centre
180 Woodbridge Street
Fredericton, NB
E3B 4R3
Tel: (506) 452 5225

QUEBEC
Montreal Neurological Institute and Hospital
3801 University St.
Montreal, QC
H3A 2B4
Dr. Daria A. Trojan, Physiatrist

Tel: (514) 398 8911
Fax: (514) 398 7371
Dr. Diane Diorio, Neurologist
Tel: (514) 398 5034
Fax: (514) 398 3972

ONTARIO
Dr. Lo, Physiatrist
West Park Healthcare Centre
82 Buttonwood Avenue
Toronto, ON
M6M 2J5
Tel: (416) 243 3600 x2122
Fax: (416) 243 8947

Dr. Lo, Physiatrist
Sunnybrook and Women's College Health Sciences Centre
2075 Bayview Ave.
Toronto, ON
M4N 3M5
Tel: (416) 480 6930
Fax: (416) 480 6585

Dr. Neil R. Cashman, Neurologist
Neuromuscular Clinic
Sunnybrook & Women's College Health Sciences Centre
2075 Bayview Ave.
Toronto, ON
M4N 3M5
Tel: (416) 480 4213
Fax: (807) 344 3891
neil.cashman@utoronto.ca

Dr. Sharma, Physiatrist
Kensington Clinic
340 College St.
Toronto, ON
M5T 3A9
Tel: (416) 603 2725

Dr. Hargadon, Physiatrist
St. Joseph's Hospital
Box 3251

Thunder Bay, ON
P7B 5G7
Tel: (807) 345 0510
Fax: (807) 344 3891

SASKATCHEWAN
Dr. Mavis Matheson, General Practitioner
Tel: (306) 586 5094
matheson@accesscomm.ca

Dr. Lila Rudachyk, Physiatrist
City Hospital
701 Queen Street - 7th Floor
Saskatoon, SK
S7K 0M7
Tel: (306) 655-8175

ALBERTA
Dr. Ming Chan, Physiatrist
Division of Physical Medicine and Rehabilitation
University of Alberta
513 Heritage Medical Research Centre
Edmonton, AB
T6G 2S2
Tel: (780) 492 1614
Fax: (780) 492 1617
ming.cnan@ualberta.ca

Dr. Evan Sampson, Physiatrist
120-11910 - 111 Avenue
Edmonton, AB
T5G 0E5
Tel: (780) 447 4924
Fax: (780) 452 5111

Dr. Steven McNeil, Physiatrist
Foothills Medical Centre
1403 29 St. N.W.
Calgary, AB
T2N 2T9
Tel: (403) 944 4224

BRITISH COLUMBIA
Post-Polio Clinic
Dr. Elizabeth Dean, Physiotherapist
M. Dallimore, Physiotherapist
School of Rehabilitation Sciences
University of British Columbia
2211 Westbrook Mall
Vancouver, BC
V6T 1Z3

G.F. Strong Rehab Centre
Dr. Andrew Travlos, Physiatrist
4255 Lurel St.
Vancouver, BC
V5Z 2G9
Tel: (604) 734 1313
Fax: (604) 737 6359

Bibliography

Black, Kathryn. *In the Shadow of Polio: A Personal and Social History*. Addison Wesley Publishing Company. Jacob Way, Reading, MA 01867, 1996.

Bruno, Richard L. *Polio Paradox. What You Need to Know*. Warner Books, 2002.

Carsley, John, MD. *Making Sense of Anti-Vaccination Literature*. Polio Folio, Vol. 2, No. 15, Winter 1995/96. ,

Cashman, Neil, MD and Daria Trojan, MD. *Current Trends in Post-Poliomyelitis Syndrome*. Milestone Medical Communications, Division of Ruder-Finn, 301 East 57th St., New York City, 1996. (An educational service of ICN Pharmaceuticals, Inc.)

Dalakas, Marinos. "Post-Polio Syndrome 12 Years Later. How It All Started." *Annals of The New York Academy of Sciences*. Vol. 753, May 25, 1995. pp. 11-18.

Davey, Sheila. *Polio: The Beginning of the End*. World Health Organization, Geneva, 1997.

Davies. B. *Death Walks in Summer*.

Frappier, Armand, MD. *Un rêve, une lutte. Autobiographie*. Presses de l'Université du Quebec, C.P. 250, Sillery, QC G1T 2R1, 1992.

Gingras, Gustave, MD. *Feet Was I to the Lame*. Human Horizons Series, A Condor Book, Souvenir Press (Educational and Academic) Ltd., Methuen Publications, Agincourt, ON.

Gould, Tony. *A Summer Plague: Polio and Its Survivors*, Yale University Press, New Haven, 1995.

Halstead, Lauro S., MD. "Post-Polio Syndrome". *Scientific American*, 1998:42-47.

Halstead, Lauro S., MD and Naomi Naierman, MPA, eds. *Managing Post-Polio: A Guide to Living Well with Post-Polio Syndrome*. NRH Press, Washington, D.C., 1998.

Health Heritage Research Services. Compiled by Christopher Rutty. http://

www.healthheritageresearch.com .

Hull, Harry. "Progress Towards the Global Eradication of Poliomyelitis." *Rehabilitation*, 4207 Lindell Boulevard, #110, St. Louis, MO, 63108-2915. Summer 1998, Vol. 38, No. 2.

Kiple, Kenneth F., ed. "Polio", in *Cambridge World History of Human Disease*. Cambridge University Press, 1993, p. 1176.

Lutwick, Larry I., MD. "Warts in the Poliosaur Bones: The Successes and Failures of Poliomyelitis Vaccines in the U.S.", *Medscape*, June 26, 1998. See web page http://www.medscape.com .

Martin, Paul. *A Very Public Life*, 2 volumes. Deneau Publishers, Ottawa. 1983, 1985.

"Monkey Virus DNA Found in Rare Human Cancers", *Science* Vol. 275, February 7, 1998.

Munsat, Theodore L., MD. *Post-Polio Syndrome*. Butterworth and Heinemann, 1991.

Polio Network News, International Polio Network, St. Louis, Missouri.

Polio Quebec's Web Page with links to many other polio and disability web sites: http://www.polioquebec.org .

Polio: The Beginning of the End, World Health Organization, Geneva, 1997.

Post-Polio Task Force, *Post-Polio Syndrome Update*, BioScience Communications, 1997.

Preston, Richard. *The Hot Zone*, Random House, 1994.

Prytula, Michael A., ND. "No Vaccines for My Kids", *Alive Magazine*, #155, 1995.

Rotarian, The. Regular updates in Rotary International's monthly magazine under the heading "Polio Plus" on the progress of their goal to eradicate polio by the year 2005 (originally the year 2000).

Rutty, Christopher J. "40 Years of Polio Prevention. Canada and the Great Salk Vaccine Trial of 1954-55", *Abilities Magazine*. Summer 1994. p. 26

Rutty, Christopher J. *Do Something!.... Do Anything! Poliomyelitis in Canada 1927-1962*. PhD Thesis, University of Toronto, Department of History, 1998.

Sass, Edmund J., MD with George Gottfried and Anthony Sorem. *Polio's Legacy: An Oral History.* University Press of America, Inc., Lanham, MD, 1996.

Silver, Julie K. MD. *Post-Polio Syndrome: A Guide for Polio Survivors and Their Families.* Yale University Press, 2001.

Smith, Jane S. *Patenting the Sun: Polio and the Salk Vaccine.* William Morrow and Co., Inc. N.Y., 1982.

Third Canadian National Immunization Conference (Dec. 6-9, 1998). Organized by the Laboratory Centre for Disease Control, Health Canada, and the Canadian Pediatric Society.

Trojan, Daria A., MD, MSc. "Post-Polio Syndrome: The Legacy of Polio". *The Canadian Journal of Diagnosis*, March 2001.

The Magazine of the World Health Organization, special issue "Towards a World without Polio". January-February 1995.

Index

About the Editors

Sally Aitken is a community activist who had polio early in childhood. She served two terms as a Westmount city councillor and is co-author of *Histoire vécu de la Polio au Québec.*

Helen D'Orazio enjoyed a 27-year-long career in nursing until she developed symptoms of post-polio syndrome. She now volunteers for the Polio Quebec Association.

Stewart Valin is a biophysicist. His father, James, had polio.

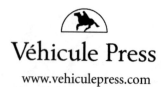

Véhicule Press
www.vehiculepress.com